RAVES FOR

THE
bloomingdale's
EAT* HEALTHY DIET

"The Bloomingdale's Eat* Healthy Diet reflects the hall-marks that make Bloomingdale's what it is. Just as Bloomingdale's is dedicated to keeping its customers up to date on the latest in fashion knowledge and style, The Bloomingdale's Eat* Healthy Diet represents the latest in nutrition and health...I encourage anyone interested in effective weight loss and maintenance to try it."

—Marvin Traub, Chairman, Bloomingdale's

"NOT ANOTHER DIET BUT A WHOLE NEW WAY OF EATING...THE WEIGHT DROPS OFF AND YOU START TO FEEL MORE ENERGETIC THAN A SIX-YEAR-OLD...IT'S NOTHING SHORT OF AMAZING!"   —Erica Jong

---

"The Bloomingdale's Eat* Healthy Diet is a winner. It focuses on the important issue of weight control, feeling good about your body, and low-fat diet and exercise. The three-staged treatment approach is just what the doctor ordered."   —George L. Blackburn, M.D., Ph.D.
                    Chief, Nutrition/Metabolism Laboratory
                    New England Deaconess Hospital, and
                    Associate Professor of Surgery, Harvard
                    Medical School

"The Bloomingdale's Eat* Healthy Diet provides you with a new beginning in personal style—one, to be beautiful and healthy; and two, to maintain these essential attributes for a lifetime."   —Brenda Vaccaro

_____

"I applaud and shout 'bravo' to a program that is as smashingly healthy as it is delicious."
                                        —Joshua Logan
                                          stage and film director

_____

"A STATE-OF-THE-ART DIET PLAN BY A HANDS-ON PRAC-TITIONER:SAFE, SANE AND SENSIBLE."   —Joseph Papp

_____

"What's so impressive is that Effective Appetite Training sets up a whole new pattern of healthy eating habits, habits that we can all live with and adapt to our life styles—while it also generates the quick weight loss that patients need to keep motivated."
                                        —Saul I. Heller, M.D.

"I had been a successful dieter my entire adult life. Laura Stein had nothing to teach me. Four weeks after starting her Eat Healthy program, she had profoundly changed my relationship with food and literally my life. I eat more food and different foods, enjoy it more than ever, guilt free, and haven't stopped losing weight. And I've never felt better."

—Barbara Griff
Television Producer

———————————

"When I started the program 12/9/84, my blood pressure was 150 over 92 and my heart rate was 96. On 2/9/85, my blood pressure was 118 over 75 and my heart rate was 68. Nothing I can say would be more dramatic than that."

—Richard Fisher
Executive

THE
bloomingdale's
EAT*HEALTHY DIET
*EFFECTIVE APPETITE TRAINING

LAURA STEIN
With Preface By
GEORGE L. BLACKBURN,
M.D., Ph.D.

ST. MARTIN'S PRESS/NEW YORK

NOTE TO THE READER:

Menus and recipes in this book have been analyzed by the Research Dietician of the Metabolic Unit of St. Lukes–Roosevelt Hospital. Of course, no diet can be ideal for every individual. Accordingly, the reader should consult with a physician before undertaking this or any other diet or exercise program. This is especially important if the reader has any medical condition or is taking any medications that might be affected by diet or exercise.

The diet and program are the result of the author's research and experience. Neither the publisher nor Bloomingdale's makes any warranty, express or implied, with respect to this book or its contents, and neither is or shall be liable for any claims arising from use of or reliance upon this book.

Copyright © 1986 by Laura Stein
Preface copyright © 1986 by George L. Blackburn, M.D., Ph.D.

All rights reserved. No part of this book may be used or reproduced in any manner whatsoever without written permission except in the case of brief quotations embodied in critical articles or reviews. For information address St. Martin's Press, 175 Fifth Avenue, New York, N. Y. 10010.

Library of Congress Catalog Card Number: 86-1279

ISBN: 0-312-90641-2   Can. ISBN: 0-312-90642-0

Printed in the United States of America

First St. Martin's Press mass market edition/January 1987

10 9 8 7 6 5 4 3 2 1

I wish to dedicate this book to everyone
who has ever awakened with the thought:
I'm really going to be good today.

Acknowledgments

I want to express my appreciation and profound gratitude to those who contributed to the development of the technique I call Appetite Training and to this book. Without their efforts, support, and confidence in me, *The Bloomingdale's Eat Healthy Diet* would never have been born.

- The Breakthrough Foundation put me in touch with my profound commitment to change the way people eat and gave me the courage and skills to take on the job.
- Danny Abraham first focused my attention on appetite and showed me the path. He's the real father of the project.
- Marvin Traub has believed in and followed the program and has been an enthusiastic proponent of the diet.
- Kate Mattias assisted me every inch of the way. Her commitment and vision were critical in making the program, the Workshop, and the book a reality.
- The late Dr. Saul I. Heller provided a sound medical

basis and confirmed my belief that I was on the right track.

- Dr. George L. Blackburn, out of his commitment to promoting good health and his belief in the program, offered invaluable insight and support.
- Sandie Woller and Joanne Kinzinger were two of my original trial dieters whose commitment and feedback were invaluable.
- My "live lab," my first Workshop participants—David Campbell, Liza Dawson, Frank Emblen, Don Karras, Kate Mattias, Mary Reilly, Jahn Snyder and Wendy Snyder, Esther Unterman, and Gene Wolsk—made it real.
- Marge Piatak blazed the Bloomingdale's trail with her superb results and contagious enthusiasm.
- Margaret Hofbeck was never too busy to listen, care, and offer wise counsel.
- Leslie Lang, Dino Yiachos, and Seth Flesher provided the research to support my theories.
- Julie Bukar, R.D., provided the research and knowledge that ensured balanced menus and recipes, and accurate nutritional information throughout.
- Mary Reilly helped demonstrate that food can be healthy, guilt-free, and delicious. Many of the recipes bear her special touch.
- Liza Dawson and Barbara Anderson, my editors, helped create order out of intermittent chaos.
- Gerry Schwartz, first my friend, also my lawyer, helped make the agreements that made everyone happy.
- Meredith Bernstein, my agent, had the dedication and insight that helped shape this book through many incarnations.
- My parents, Sylvia and Joe Stein, always told me I could do it, whatever "it" was. They also taught me that food was one of life's great pleasures and therefore a worthy obsession.
- Gene Wolsk was my toughest test case and is my most passionate supporter.

Contents

Foreword

Innovation. Creativity. Energy. Vitality. These are traditions at Bloomingdale's—the trademarks that give us the competitive edge in retailing—the ingredients that generate the electricity that vibrates in every area of our stores.

The Bloomingdale's Eat Healthy Diet reflects the hallmarks that make Bloomingdale's what it is. Just as Bloomingdale's is dedicated to keeping its customers up to date on the latest in fashion knowledge and style, *The Bloomingdale's Eat Healthy Diet* represents the latest in nutrition and health. Here is a diet that will help you lose weight by eating healthy foods that taste great, look great . . . and give you that winning edge of energy and vitality.

In fact, it is this energy and vitality that first brought the diet to my attention. I noticed that an unusual number of our top executives were losing weight. And they all seemed disturbingly cheerful about the process. They had been attending the New York-based Eat Healthy Workshop, originated by Laura Stein. I was surrounded by a new breed of evangelist—fitness evangelists.

I discussed this growing phenomenon with my wife, Lee, one evening and we decided to give the diet a try. The Eat Healthy Workshop that we attended began on January 10, 1985. By the final session, five weeks later, I had lost fifteen pounds, only four pounds short of my ultimate goal, which I reached a few weeks after that.

Changing the balance of the foods I ate improved how I looked and felt. It also enhanced my sense of well-being. The best part of all was that I gratefully embraced the process.

I was convinced that the benefits I'd derived from the program were significant. And I saw my own experience mirrored in those around me. In the spring of '85 we added it up and discovered that the thirty-three of us at Bloomingdale's who had completed Laura Stein's Eat Healthy Workshop had lost over five hundred pounds. Since many had followed the program more for its health benefits and Appetite Training than for weight loss, the average loss of sixteen pounds was even more impressive. One notable aspect of the Eat Healthy experience was the *esprit de corps* we shared as a result of our common commitment.

The interest of Bloomingdale's executives in Eat Healthy was so profound that those who work with us began to refer to the program as "the Bloomingdale's diet." I began to hear the message. I wanted to enhance the positive reactions that were already apparent, so we have offered participation in Laura Stein's Eat Healthy Workshop as a part of the Bloomingdale's executive benefit program. After all, Bloomingdale's employees are a reflection of Bloomingdale's customers. If we had embraced the Eat Healthy method for weight loss and Effective Appetite Training, those who shared our lifestyle and concerns would want to as well. Thus, Bloomingdale's has joined forces with Laura Stein, creator of the Eat Healthy method, and we offer you *The Bloomingdale's Eat Healthy Diet.*

The Bloomingdale's Eat Healthy Diet is an extraordinary experience. It is a positive program that reflects the human desire to enjoy the sense of taste, yet create a personal image that is self enhancing. We believe this diet can provide you with the same vitality, energy, and exuberance that we seek to convey to our customers. We suggest that Effective Appetite Training, because of its lasting values, may be one of the most positive experiences of your life.

At this writing, I've now been in the Personalization phase of The Bloomingdale's Eat Healthy Diet for almost six months. I have not regained the nineteen pounds I lost. I find I still enjoy good food, feel satisfied after most meals, and am very happy with my new weight. I believe I am healthier on The Bloomingdale's Eat Healthy Diet and I encourage anyone interested in effective weight loss and maintenance to try it.

—Marvin Traub
Chairman, Bloomingdale's

Preface

The key to successful weight control is developing pleasure in eating while ridding the body of excess fat. The goal is to develop a new lifestyle where eating, exercise, daily planning, and stress management result in maintaining a natural body size that is healthy and supportive of personal goals and quality of life. But while the goal is clear, many people are unsure about how to start—and maintain—such a program. *The Bloomingdale's Eat Healthy Diet,* with its three-staged approach, is an ideal way to get started on the road to a healthful way of eating. It focuses on important issues of weight control, such as feeling good about your body, appetite control, low-fat diet, and exercise. It is a medically sound program that, without requiring a crash diet or a faddish way of eating, will help bring weight down to a sensible level and at the same time help reduce the intake of cholesterol, sodium, and fat.

The dietary advice given in *The Bloomingdale's Eat Healthy Diet* is consistent with the latest findings of the medical community. Recently, the obesity nutrition scientific community at the National Institutes of Health (NIH) developed a consensus on exactly what obesity is (primarily development of excess body fat), and what the consequences of an obese condition are (increased risk of physical and mental illness and loss of the quality of life). Also, the North American Association for the Study of Obesity as well as other major federal agencies have identified the desirable weight-loss characteristics of a low-fat diet. These include consuming food in moderation and eating less fat and more complex carbohydrate (high fiber/roughage food). The American Cancer Society, the American Heart Association, the American Diabetes Society, and the American Dietetic Association similarly have endorsed these dieting guidelines.

Indeed, "therapeutic diets" focused on low fat intake for treatment of breast cancer and colon cancer using multicenter trials sponsored by the National Cancer Institute. Dietary treatment of high blood pressure in the overweight and obese is supported by the National Heart Lung and Blood Institute. A variety of other diet and nutrition programs of interest to all Americans is coordinated by the Nutrition Committee at the National Institutes of Health.

Also endorsed is the multidisciplinary approach to weight control combining diet and nutrition with behavior and exercise programs to effect the required lifestyle change. A highly recommended exercise is walking or an equivalent effort that would sustain expenditure of 2,000 calories per week. This usually takes three to four hours per week to accomplish. These thirty- to sixty-minute brisk walks three to four times per week should be combined with behavior programs aimed at planning, relaxing, coping, and managing the routine mental stresses of daily living.

Laura Stein developed the Eat Healthy program from her personal research on nutrition. After extensive experience in her Eat Healthy Workshops, she translated this experience into *The Bloomingdale's Eat Healthy Diet*. The Eat Healthy

Workshops provide a human laboratory to support her assertion and methods for diet and weight control.

Laura Stein has produced a plan that works. Her approach calls for eating food that is not only tasty, but that also triggers the digestive tract and naturally resulting metabolism to produce a feeling of fullness and relief of hunger. These are essential to a successful weight-control program. Laura Stein has divided her program into three phases—Transition, Stabilization, and Personalization—an approach that is consistent with the best principles of behavior change. Professor Emeritus B. F. Skinner, a noted Harvard behavior scientist, emphasized avoidance of unwanted behavior and substitution of desirable behavior to fill this void as the cornerstone of behavior change activity. The Transition phase of *The Bloomingdale's Eat Healthy Diet* is an effective means of achieving this objective. During this stage, cravings for sweet, salty, and fatty foods can be replaced with cravings for healthy food.

The Bloomingdale's Eat Healthy Diet produces a change in the way you experience the taste and texture of your usual foods. Some people will find this takes time, particularly because of the increased fiber and roughage of the diet. Certain individuals with irritable bowel or digestive disorders may require a consultation with their physician. As with the treatment of many conditions, the outcome will depend upon the effort and motivation of the individual. Compliance to the details of the diet produce the best results. The quantity of food consumed, speed of eating, and the amount of chewing all affect the satisfaction of eating and the tolerance of your digestive tract. As with any weight-loss program, supplementation with a simple vitamin/mineral pill (particularly one containing zinc, selenium, magnesium, iron, and calcium) ensures intake of essential micronutrients.

In summary, *The Bloomingdale's Eat Healthy Diet* is an essential first step to a sensible, prudent, safe, and effective diet program. It provides the essential elements for achieving a desirable body size and a personal lifestyle aimed at a high quality of life with a low risk for diet-related illness. When necessary or desirable, you can incorporate the program within your family setting, self-help groups, and adult education seminars, and in consultation with registered dietitians specializing in therapeutic diets, and with your physician.

The Bloomingdale's Eat Healthy Diet is a winner. It is just what a doctor would order for healthy patients and desirable eating habits.

—George L. Blackburn, M.D., Ph.D.
Chief, Nutrition/Metabolism Laboratory,
New England Deaconess Hospital, and
Associate Professor of Surgery,
Harvard Medical School

Resources for Further Information

- "Health Implications of Obesity," 1985. Office of Medical Applications of Research, Building 1, Room 216, National Institutes of Health, Bethesda, Maryland 20205.
- U.S. Government Printing Office pamphlet "Dietary Guidelines for Americans," 2nd edition, 1985. U.S. Department of Agriculture/U.S. Department of Health and Human Services. Home and Garden Bulletin #232.
- North American Association for the Study of Obesity (NAASO), c/o Mario DeGirolamo, M.D., President, Emory University School of Medicine, Atlanta, Georgia 30303.
- Nutrition Coordinating Committee, Office of the Director, Building 1, National Institutes of Health, Bethesda, Maryland 20205.
- *Recent Advances in Obesity Research: IV,* Jules Hirsch and Theodore B. Van Itallie, editors, 1985, John Libbey & Co., Ltd., London, England.

Introduction

• Jane had been fashionably thin all her life and had never needed to worry about what she ate. But now, approaching thirty, she was steadily gaining weight and was unable to control her eating. Suddenly she understood why the rest of the world was diet crazy. Thirty extra pounds padded her body; she was terrified that she was out of control and would never look like her "normal" self again.

• Rebecca didn't have much sympathy for Jane's problem. Rebecca had never had the luxury of indulging without gaining weight. She'd been a fat child, a fat teenager, a fat young mother, and now, at the age of forty-five, she was seventy pounds overweight. She had given up on herself, becoming resigned to a lifetime of half-sizes and a miserable, self-conscious distaste for all social situations.

• Dennis was a beef-and-gravy-loving former football player who looked anything but athletic as his 5'11" frame tipped the scales at 240 pounds. His wife found big men attractive. That suited him just fine. Then his doctor convinced him that, with his medical history, he was courting a heart attack if he didn't radically alter his eating habits and lose fifty pounds. He assumed that once he set his mind to it he wouldn't have much trouble losing the weight. His confidence was rocked, however, as he found himself depressed, gaining weight instead of losing it, and unable to control his now escalating appetite.

• No one would ever suspect that Melanie had a diet problem. As an eighteen-year-old college freshman, Melanie had the body of a model. But she knew that her self-devised method for staying slim was taking its toll. In order to allow herself the sugary snacks she craved, she cut calories by not eating other, more nutritious foods. She avoided restaurants and meals with friends because she didn't want to "waste" the calories. She preferred staying home and binging on cookies and candy bars. Sometimes she ate to the point of nausea. Recently this was occuring more often, and Melanie was afraid she was losing control.

What all these people have in common is a problem with food and dieting. But today their lives are different. Each discovered a profound new resource that allowed them to end a history of diet failure and break the destructive habits that had caused them so much pain.

What made the difference? The answer is simple: They learned how to train their appetites so they would crave food that contributed to a slim, healthy body. They each conquered the persistent cravings and defeating habits that had kept them from having the bodies they wanted—not by denying themselves the food they loved, but by *altering their desires so that they could eat as a reward and not a punishment*. What they learned was that they could love food and still be thin. The result was not only a dramatic and permanent weight loss, but also a new love and appreciation of healthy food. They became free of the turmoil and conflict they had once experienced. And that's exactly what I'm going to teach you. Everything you need to know to train your own appetite and establish a positive relationship with food is in this book.

My appetite was trained over years of struggling with my own weight problem. I'd gained weight as an adolescent and suffered with the conflicts that result from the vicious cycle of being overweight. Every morning I'd wake up and promise myself I was going to be "good." At some point during the day I'd break that promise when some craving was stronger than my good intentions. It caused me years of frustration and misery. I am 5'5" and at my heaviest I weighed 150 pounds. It might as well have been double that for all the time and attention I devoted to the problem. Weight was the controlling issue of my life. Everything in those years revolved around what I did or didn't, could or couldn't eat.

As I grew older the problem intensified because I went to work in the fashion and beauty business. I became the marketing editor of *Vogue* magazine, and then held top corporate positions at Elizabeth Arden and Chanel. I recognized that I had to control the problem in order to compete effectively in my industry. How you looked, how you "packaged" yourself, was critical to your success. Career advancement was a powerful motivator, but I was still only intermittently successful with my diets. I managed to take off fifteen of the thirty pounds I needed to lose, but I yo-yo'ed up and down with the last fifteen.

It was after I started my own business and began working professionally in the diet industry that I learned firsthand what works and what doesn't when you're trying to lose weight. Studying the subject helped me reorient my approach from a negative one, in which I felt sorry for myself because I had a weight problem, to a positive one in which I took an active interest in the role food played in preventive medicine and in promoting good health. I worked as a consultant on developing new diets and diet products, and on research with existing diet programs and diet aids. I wrote magazine articles on dieting, nutrition, and fitness for *Family Circle, Ladies' Home Journal, Prevention,* and *Cosmopolitan.* All the while, I was involved with the real experts on the subject: the dieters themselves.

I saw that it was a fortunate minority who genuinely conquered their weight problem. Most of the men and women involved in the projects on which I was working, or whom I interviewed for research and articles, fit the classic pattern. That is, even though they had been successful in losing weight, they invariably gained it back, most often regaining slightly more than they had lost.

I wondered what separated the successful dieters from everyone else. The difference that eventually became clear to me was that those who were able to maintain their weight loss were those who were able to establish a new relationship with food. They had learned to enjoy food—and to stop punishing themselves with it. They had been able to give up the idea that they were missing something because they had stopped routinely eating those foods that had made them fat. I realized that what was needed was a mechanism that could give someone the ability to establish that new relationship. I was convinced that that was the key to success.

There was one other, ever-present characteristic in the successful dieters: they had all integrated exercise into their lives. They all included exercise as a desirable part of their day.

It became evident that the problem was not one of losing weight but one of *maintaining* a weight loss. I saw over and over again that people are great dieters. It almost seemed irrelevant what diet they chose. Once committed, people tend to be faithful to a diet for some amount of time. And that's the problem with most diets. They concentrate on short-term weight loss, not the long-term reality of relating to food.

The truth is that no matter what specific quirks you like or dislike about any given diet, no diet in the world can help you lose weight permanently until you learn to control your appetite, and not let it control you. Traditional diets do not make any long-term changes in your appetite. If you continue to crave the foods of your undoing, you're destined for a future no different from your past.

All of this became clear as I concentrated on the distinction between successful and failed dieters. In 1981, I began to experiment with various methods of producing an actual change in appetite response. Problem dieters tended to be dependent on overly sweet and salty tastes, as well as on high-fat food. Those who eventually established new habits managed to cut those dependencies. I was well aware that people with high blood pressure had little trouble living on a low-salt diet once they'd made the initial adjustment. Those who had managed to kick the sugar habit reported a similar experience. And it's also common for red-meat lovers who have heeded recommendations to cut their consumption to report that they miss meat less and less as time goes by. But for most people, the common methods of cutting down don't work. They may make inroads in one area, only to find their progress undermined by runaway cravings in another.

Slowly, with the help of a variety of willing subjects, I formulated a program that actually conquered cravings by reintroducing people to food. The most successful strategy became the basis for a ten-day plan that I now call the Transition phase. A version of this approach was published as the Purification Diet in the *Ladies' Home Journal* in 1983. It worked to produce a dramatic weight loss while it effectively cut problematic food addictions. This staged reintroduction to food allowed people to become used to a new balance of food in their meals, one more in keeping with the most recent nutritional thinking, which emphasizes complex carbohydrates, not protein and fat.

The incredible results that this process generated convinced me that I was on the right track. Sweetaholics told me they were amazed at how painless cutting out sweets had been. Going "cold turkey," it seemed, had been easier than trying to cut down. The initial thought might have been that they could live through anything for ten days as long as it produced a significant weight loss, but the experience had actually been pleasant! People reported having increased energy, instead of the lethargy they associated with dieting. And, most encouraging of all, they were asking for what to do next. They wanted to stay with the program. They wanted advice for a sustained regimen that followed similar principles.

The ten-day program had produced exactly what I'd hoped: It had given people the experience of a new relationship with food. It had reintroduced them to flavor and texture so they could appreciate what they were eating. Dieters reported that they found themselves craving the next food group the day before they were allowed to eat it. So they had the experience of craving bread instead of cake, chicken instead of pizza. Now what was necessary was to outline an ongoing program that gave people enough time to solidify this new experience. One more effective diet wouldn't make a difference. What was genuinely wanted and needed was a new philosophy of eating.

I knew that people loved food and wanted to be able to enjoy its pleasures. Any program that tried to ignore this simple reality was bound to fail. My long-term strategy, therefore, had to concentrate on eating, not dieting.

To help me gain insight into the complex patterns of the ongoing process, I put together a group of dieters to give me more experience with the nuances of Appetite Training. These men and women agreed to meet together with me for five weeks as a "live laboratory." What we discovered, I synthesized into three phases that I called Transition, Stabilization, and Personalization. Without exception, people needed the impact of the intensive ten-day, quick weight-loss, Appetite Training phase (Transition); then a period to let their new habits genuinely take hold while they continued to lose weight (Stabilization); and, finally, they needed to be able to establish a relationship with food that allowed them to include indulgences when they wanted them, without letting those indulgences become the bad habits they once were (Personalization).

The results were astonishing, even to me. In addition to impressive weight losses—which ranged from seven pounds for a few women who didn't have much to lose, to more than twenty pounds for several men and women who were heavier—the benefits seemed too good to be true. As I mentioned before, increased energy was a major factor for most participants. Fewer mood swings and improved skin conditions were also noted by some. But what couldn't have been anticipated was the incredible sense of well-being and confidence that permeated the group. And it was noticeable. Friends of my original live laboratory began to ask me if I needed more human guinea pigs on whom to experiment. The requests became so commonplace that Eat Healthy Workshops (EAT stands for Effective Appetite Training) were born. I've been conducting Eat Healthy Workshops ever since—and refining the program in the process.

The last chapter in the story of the evolution of Eat Healthy is the one in which the program was discovered and adopted by Bloomingdale's. It began when Marge Piatak, Director of Wage and Salary Planning for the store, lost thirty-five pounds in the Workshop. Her success and enthusiasm caused others who worked with her to attend our Workshops. Slowly, the Eat Healthy Workshop became the "in" thing to do in an organization devoted to discovering the latest trends. What none of us were prepared for were the additional benefits that surfaced once the Bloomingdale's Eat Healthy team grew in number. Not only did the many executives who had completed the program reinforce and support each other, but the positive feelings they derived from eating well and accomplishing such important personal goals seemed to have a ripple effect that fostered an unusual *esprit de corps.*

When Bloomingdale's chairman, Marvin Traub, lost fifteen pounds in his Eat Healthy Workshop, he became convinced that our method of Effective Appetite Training was dramatically different and could make a meaningful contribution to Bloomingdale's customers as well as its employees. What was most impressive was that the program worked for a group of retailing professionals—no small feat, in an industry where twelve-hour days and frequent domestic and foreign travel are commonplace.

So, Bloomingdale's established an ongoing relationship with us, first by making the Eat Healthy plan available to the store's executive employees through a corporate benefits plan, and then by bringing us to a wider public in the form of this book.

The program put forward in *The Bloomingdale's Eat Healthy Diet* is a well-tested one. I've watched it work successfully for a wide variety of men and women since I began experimenting with it in 1981. What's more, I've seen that the results not only last, but also increase over time. The most gratifying thing for me has been the overwhelming commitment to Eat Healthy that's been demonstrated by Workshop participants. The stories that opened this introduction are only a few of the many I'll refer to in these pages. Seeing someone like Rebecca conquer a lifelong weight problem makes me feel like my own version of Rocky. I consider myself an unusually lucky person to be able to interact with people in a way that makes such a difference to them. Knowing that Eat Healthy enables people to realize their most profound dreams and aspirations regarding their one and only body is the greatest reward I can imagine.

—Laura Stein

The Basics of
The Bloomingdale's Eat Healthy Diet

What Is *The Bloomingdale's Eat Healthy Diet?*

The Bloomingdale's Eat Healthy Diet is a new philosophy of healthful eating that contributes to fast, permanent weight loss through its exclusive method of Effective Appetite Training. It is a three-phase program that gives you all the tools you need to establish a new and rewarding relationship with food. Specifically, the three phases are:

Transition. The first phase of Appetite Training, this ten-day regimen makes your digestive system feel cleansed, cuts your food addictions, and promotes a substantial, initial weight loss. Most people lose between five and twelve pounds in the ten-day Transition period alone—eating delicious food the whole time. During the Transition phase you are returned to your natural appetite response by progressively reintroducing yourself to each food group.

You begin by eating vegetables, then add grains, poultry and fish, dairy products, and fruit on subsequent days. The timing of the reintroduction of each food group is strategically aimed at allowing you to appreciate its special qualities while maximizing your weight loss. You will anticipate the flavors and nuances of texture of each category of food before you get to add it. This staged reintroduction works to focus your attention away from the foods you currently crave and onto those that form the basis of the *The Bloomingdale's Eat Healthy Diet*. By the end of the first week you are eating a well-rounded, delicious, nutritionally balanced diet while you enjoy fast weight-loss results.

One of the unexpected benefits of the Transition phase is that because you are not eating extremely sweet and salty food, your tastebuds become more sensitive to a wider range of flavors. Our tastebuds can distinguish only sweet, salty, sour, and bitter. The more you flood your palate with sweet and salty sensations, the less sensitive it becomes. In Transition you begin truly to taste food again and a whole new realm of eating pleasure is opened up to you.

Stabilization. The second phase of *The Bloomingdale's Eat Healthy Diet*, Stabilization, allows you to continue to lose weight steadily while you learn to accommodate a new balance of foods in your diet, one in keeping with the latest nutritional thinking. During Stabilization you have an opportunity to indulge your new cravings as you concentrate on the positive approach to fast weight loss. The emphasis now is on eating. After all, why diet when you can eat—and still lose weight in the process?

The foods that form the mainstay of your diet during Stabilization include many of those formerly thought to be fattening. Potatoes, rice, pasta, bread, and crackers are now part of your everyday meals, besides vegetables, fruits, dairy products, poultry, meat, and fish. The recipes and cooking strategies in Chapter 8 offer enticing suggestions and a variety of ingenious cooking techniques that encourage you to fully explore your new positive preoccupation with food. In addition, there is lots of helpful advice for eating out and socializing.

The other aspect of the Stabilization phase is its attention to the stimulus/response patterns that govern eating habits. Now that your physical appetite is satisfied, you can address the more emotional and instinctive reasons you eat. This phase enables you to deal realistically with the complex behavior patterns that have been the source of past diet failures. The result is a new self-confidence around food that lets you enjoy its pleasures without being undermined by old destructive habits.

Stabilization is your blueprint for a lifetime of happy, healthy eating. Learning to channel the negative energy that you've expended on failing to lose weight into a positive outlet that concentrates on eating to lose weight is nothing short of miraculous. As you will see in Chapter 2, there is a difference between a "fat" and "thin" mentality regarding food. To think that you will ever be thin through restraint is to believe that you can totally change your basic nature. Perhaps this is theoretically possible, but I've yet to see it happen. Instead, Stabilization teaches you that the only way to be thin is to capitalize on your love of food. It's a sensualist's approach to losing weight.

Personalization. Personalization begins after you reach your goal. It's the phase of Appetite Training that takes into consideration each person's individual preferences. The truth is that none of us wants to deny himself or herself whole categories of food. When your natural appetite response is operating, you will discover that you crave your old downfalls much less than you do now. But who wants to go through life without pizza or pastrami? Similarly, a delicious dessert doesn't have to make you feel guilty. The key is to be able to love your indulgences, not suffer from them.

By the time you are in Personalization you will know the difference between real cravings and what I call "reflexive" cravings. This important distinction is what will enable you to obtain the right balance of those foods that must be limited in order not to regain your weight or undermine the effectiveness of your Appetite Training. You will be surprised, by the way, to discover which foods it is that you genuinely miss —and how rarely you miss them. What's critical to know is that when you do miss them, you should eat them. The beauty of Personalization is that it is totally up to you.

The three-phase process of *The Bloomingdale's Eat Healthy Diet* is so effective that you will be able to trust yourself with this much freedom of choice. Your new relationship to food is firmly established only when you choose it as a preference after you are thin. What you'll be delighted to discover is how automatic that choice becomes.

Why Does *The Bloomingdale's Eat Healthy Diet* Work?

The Bloomingdale's Eat Healthy Diet works because it has the three most important elements for your success:

1. *The weight comes off fast.* Rapid weight loss is great for your morale. It may be sensible to lose weight slowly, but it often takes more discipline than you have to stick with it. Because of the way Transition is structured, some people have reported losing as much weight as they have on juice fasts, even though Transition includes filling and delicious meals. When you enter the Stabilization phase, you'll continue to lose at an amazingly steady pace.

2. *You're eating great food the whole time you're losing.* If you're not happy with the food on a diet, you'll go back to your old favorites as soon as your weight comes off, if not before. If you like the food, but it's not nutritionally balanced, you'll begin to be troubled by strong cravings. *The Bloomingdale's Eat Healthy Diet* not only offers you a wide variety of delicious, nutritionally balanced foods, but also increases your pleasure by retraining your tastebuds, along with your appetite.

3. *It addresses the emotional and habitual as well as the physical aspects of appetite.* When you have a sugar or salt habit, you crave sweet or salty foods whether you're happy or sad, calm or nervous. When your physical addictions are cured, however, and your natural appetite is genuinely satisfied, you can see your stimulus/response eating patterns more clearly. Only then can you take advantage of the techniques offered for breaking the habits that break your diet. Unless these patterns begin to break up, you're destined to gain back any weight you lose. What's fascinating is that once you begin the habit-breaking process, it tends to accelerate naturally, without much effort on your part.

What Do You Need to Succeed?

This time the magic number is five. The keys to success are commitment, food, water, exercise, and support. So let's take them one by one:

1. Commitment. Appetite Training is a bit of a roller coaster; it's an exciting ride with lots of highs and a few inevitable lows. Once you're strapped into a roller coaster car, you don't have the option of getting off until the ride is over. You need to approach Appetite Training the same way.

You need to make a commitment that's so solid that you stay on the ride, even as you go around the curves. To help you make that commitment, I want you to consider the following:

What if, instead of reading this book, you could suddenly stop craving all the things you know are "bad" for you, simply by magic. You wouldn't have to give up your cravings altogether, but instead of wanting ice cream on a hot day, you'd find yourself swooning for just a ripe wedge of honeydew melon. And in winter, a bowl of steaming vegetable soup would actually satisfy you more than a cup of hot cocoa ever could. Would you be willing to entertain the prospect?

The fascinating thing is that if you're like most people, your answer won't be an instant yes. Right now your heart is probably somewhere around your ankles. Tell the truth. You want to want ————. (You can fill in your own pet downfall here. You may hate ice cream, and crave sausages and peppers.) You don't want to give up anything you love. The reason is simple—you're human!

So now imagine that by some wave of a wand you wouldn't really miss the "goodies" (or "baddies," depending on your point of view). What's more, you'd get to crave a whole new array of enticements—foods you'd look forward to eating, the way you do ice cream now. Would you be willing? If honeydew could turn you on the way ice cream does?

The real question is, are you willing to be thin? You need to examine the paradox in your life. As much as you'd "give anything" to have the body you dream about, you qualify the "anything" when it involves your favorite foods. Yet you know that stopping bad habits for short periods of time doesn't work, not if what you want is to lose weight permanently.

Effective Appetite Training works. There's a leap of faith you need to make to prove it to yourself. You won't have to stick with Transition for long to discover that everything I'm promising is actually true. In Eat Healthy Workshops there's an atmosphere of real euphoria at the second session, after participants have been on the program for five or six days. As Dennis, who was a real skeptic, put it, "I can't believe this. I'm not hungry. I'm not craving anything. I feel terrific. Something's screwy!"

What was screwy was that his assumptions about what he needed to feel satisfied had been challenged. He was feeling great on a diet that he'd assumed was going to make him feel deprived. What's important is that he had been willing to make a commitment to explore Appetite Training for himself, even though he was skeptical. He took a leap of faith because he decided it was time to get off the fence. He was fifty-two and he knew it was only going to get harder. His doctor wasn't going to give him different advice at his next checkup. Dennis said he was willing to try anything—even if it meant joining the fitness bandwagon—if it might help him live longer and if it would reverse the unmistakable outward progression of notches on his belt.

At some point, you're going to have to make a similar leap of faith. You have to decide that this is the time for you; that you are ready to be thin. What's so exciting is that once you make the decision, once you simply say "yes" to a thin you, the result of that decision is only a matter of time. Because *The Bloomingdale's Eat Healthy Diet* is so effective, you can be closer to your goal, beginning tomorrow—as long as you follow the other four keys to success.

2. Food. As odd as it may sound, food is an essential ingredient for success. You ate your way into this problem and you're going to have to eat your way out of it. Ironically, abstaining from food won't solve anything. Sure, you'll lose weight. But if what you want is to be thin for life, you've got to learn to eat.

My experience with dieters has convinced me that binge eaters are likely to be binge dieters, that people who tend to be obsessive in one direction are just as likely to be obsessive in the other. You know the syndrome: When she's good she's very, very good, but when she's bad, she's rotten. There's an all-or-nothing approach that characterizes the way most people behave on a diet.

To achieve long-term success with Appetite Training, you have to follow the rules and eat everything you're supposed to eat. The trap is that people think that less must be better. It's not. There's a lot of food recommended on the program. You need to eat it. You need to be satisfied, not only emotionally, but physically. Food is a very important source of satisfaction. Don't deprive yourself of it unnecessarily.

3. Water. The Transition phase calls for drinking six to eight eight-ounce glasses of water every day. This is essential for success. It not only serves to keep you feeling full, but also facilitates the final stage of digestion, which is elimination. In addition, some experts believe that people often eat because they are thirsty. Water will keep you well hydrated and may supress your appetite. (NOTE: If you're epileptic, ask your physician how much water you can safely drink and follow his advice.)

Some people find it hard to drink so much liquid. Others simply forget. Don't ignore this rule. There's no way for me to emphasize enough how crucial drinking water is to the success of the program. It's also one habit that's worth cultivating. Drinking water gives you something to do. It keeps your hands and your mouth occupied. And it enhances your weight loss.

4. Exercise. Chapter 3 deals with the benefits of a sustained exercise program and how to go about beginning one. For now, I just want to remind you that I've worked with thousands of dieters and I've yet to see anyone maintain a significant weight loss, for an extended period of time, who didn't integrate exercise into his or her life.

The catch, of course, is that overweight people are often the most resistant to exercise. If you've been sedentary for a long time you may feel awkward and self-conscious about donning running shorts or a leotard and getting active. Don't be concerned. The Transition phase includes a walking regimen to get you started. And once you begin, the benefits will provide the motivation you need to continue.

Some medical experts feel that exercise works to increase your metabolic rate, which helps you burn calories faster. When you pair vigorous exercise with diet, your body has to go into its fat reserves to get the additional energy required to keep up the increased level of activity. It's estimated that a forty-five-minute workout will burn anywhere from 200 to 400 calories, depending on the level of exertion. It's like getting lunch "free." In addition, some recent studies show that you continue to burn calories at an increased rate for fifteen to twenty-four hours after you exercise. Not a bad deal when you consider that exercise also reduces hunger, improves your cardiovascular system, and acts as a natural tranquilizer.

So, if what you're after is fast, permanent weight loss, one thing you need for success is exercise. What you can't anticipate now is how much you'll look forward to it—once you take the plunge.

5. Support.   One lesson I've learned from the Workshop is that there's an immeasurable benefit from the support of being in a group. We enhance the effect by teaming up participants as "buddies" in the first session. Most people feel a bit uncomfortable with this throwback to grade school but they quickly get over it when they see how great it is to call a buddy between sessions and share experiences with someone who can empathize.

You should borrow this support technique for yourself. Create your own buddy system and use it to support your success. If possible, go on the program with a friend—or ask someone not on the program with you to act as a support person. The important thing is to choose someone who will encourage you and who won't be seduced by excuses. You want a sergeant who'll tell you that a walk in the rain will be good for you. Check in with your buddy frequently, at least three times a week. Use him or her to talk through problems or figure out answers to your questions.

Your buddy is one more way to reaffirm your commitment. Sometimes it's easier to disappoint yourself than a friend. When you increase the number of people who have a stake in your success, you help ensure it.

It's very important, as you go through the program, to keep reminding yourself of the critical five: commitment, food, water, exercise, and support. If your weight loss is stalled, or if you feel shaky for any reason, just repeat those five words. One of them is undoubtedly the source of your problem. As you say them to yourself you'll provide the clues you need to locate what's missing. Your commitment will keep you faithful, even when you feel low. The right food, and enough food, will keep you feeling satisfied and energetic. Sufficient water ensures satiety and proper hydration. Exercise will speed your weight loss and will probably improve the quality and length of your life. Finally, a buddy will give you the support of someone who cares enough to keep your best interests a priority. Together, they are the five keys to your success.

How Do You Know You Won't Fail?

As you read about the key elements for success, you might have thought to yourself that I was leaving out one very important factor—you. If you're like the majority of dieters with whom I work, you probably have some misgivings about your ability to follow through on your commitment if, or when, you make it. You undoubtedly have your own history of diet failure that makes you leery of feeling optimistic about undertaking a new program. It's like being afraid of a new love affair after you've been broken-hearted.

It's perfectly natural to have doubts. But don't let them influence your determination to achieve your goal. After all, life wouldn't be much fun if you didn't let yourself fall in love. And you'll never be thin if you aren't willing to take a risk. Just as Dennis was willing to have faith in the program —even though he was skeptical—you need to have faith in yourself, even though you may have given in to temptation in the past.

The difference this time is that you have a program to follow that is not only proven effective, but also realistic. As you read this book you will see that every possible contingency has been anticipated. I've been through the program with so many people in Eat Healthy Workshops that I've seen the pitfalls, and have had lots of experience in working them out. If the buyers at Bloomingdale's, who routinely travel to Milan, Paris, Tokyo, and London, find the program flexible enough for them, so will you. Believe me, they are human just the way you are. I'm not a Pollyanna about what's involved in the process. I'm optimistic and encouraging because I know Appetite Training works. And I know how to help ensure your success by alerting you to potential problem spots. I also know that as much as you love ice cream, you're going to love your new body more. You're going to be able to stay with *The Bloomingdale's Eat Healthy Diet* even though other diets failed you because the program is elastic, but doesn't give too much. The Personalization phase is unique. By the time you reach it, you will have a new self-confidence around food that you can't even begin to imagine now.

So you need to be willing to have faith in the program— and faith in yourself. In fact, you'll have a whole new perspective very early on in the Transition phase, which will confirm to you that your faith is justified. And, when you think about it, the only thing you have to lose is weight!

2

Creating an Appetite
for a Better Body

Food, glorious food—the pleasure and bane of our existence. It brightens our days with its sensuous delights. It darkens our nights with the thought that a spreading waistline or bulging hips won't disappear without having to deprive ourselves of its delicious comforts.

One way or another, we spend an inordinate amount of time thinking about food. It may be tempting to believe that you can change that reality for yourself; that food can become less important to you. But as you will see in this chapter, that isn't the likely solution to your problem. Some people do care about food more than others. And, I'd bet that if you're reading this book you're one of them. A much more realistic approach is to change the food you care about: Learn to crave the food that makes you thin.

Understanding Your Appetite Response

All that stands between you and the body you dream about is your appetite, and your decision to do something about it. It's that simple. Appetites change. They develop. They grow and diminish. An appetite is not an enemy to be feared. An appetite is a pleasure worth cultivating.

The Bloomingdale's Eat Healthy Diet will give you the expertise to direct your appetite. It makes it possible for you to convert from an unhealthy appetite to a healthy one that actively contributes to your weight-loss success. You'll discover that instead of craving foods that create unwanted body fat, you'll develop strong desires for those foods that contribute to the "ideal body image" you're going to create for yourself before you begin the Transition phase.

The results of this appetite conversion begin to show immediately. Instead of using food as the subtle (or not so subtle) form of punishment it is for you now, you'll enjoy food as the sensuous pleasure it's meant to be. Appetite Training allows you to treat food as a major source of joy in life, something it really can't be when eating is accompanied by guilt. But first, you have to understand the various elements that contribute to your own appetite response.

It's not uncommon to feel genuine anxiety at the prospect of denying one's "natural appetite" for some food or other. Individuals report rapid heartbeat, "butterfly" feelings in the stomach, sweating, and all sorts of anxiety-produced symptoms when they contemplate saying "no" to a strong craving.

"The way I behaved was incredible," Dorothy, a fifty-three-year-old Workshop graduate who lost forty pounds, told us one night in a support group meeting. "I used to stock up the house like we might be attacked and I wouldn't be able to get to a supermarket for months. I'd actually feel insecure—panicked, really—if I didn't have all my favorites on hand, just in case. In case of what? I wonder now."

Obviously, with so much food on hand, Dorothy could activate a craving just by opening a cabinet, refrigerator, or freezer door—which leads to another important aspect of appetite response.

Most people consume thousands of calories in mindless chewing, eating great quantities of food they neither enjoy nor benefit from physically. It's the automatic eating that you hardly notice—polishing off a basket of rolls before dinner is even served, or the food you consume hanging on to the refrigerator door while you wonder what you really feel like eating. It's what I call "reflexive" eating—the eating you do out of habit, rather than hunger.

It's important to examine the difference between physical and reflexive cravings because learning to distinguish between the two is an essential tool of *The Bloomingdale's Eat Healthy Diet.* It's not that you need to conquer your reflexive eating, either. There are those who believe that the secret to weight loss is behavior modification. I certainly think that some behavior modification techniques are useful, and will recommend them as we go along. Research indicates, however, that the fat and the thin among us behave very differently around food. Many experiences are so ingrained that you're better off accommodating your own basic nature than trying, however valiantly, to alter it fundamentally.

If you're old enough to read, you're old enough to have learned that life isn't fair. One of the most maddening inequities with which many of us have to contend is that some of us are naturally thin, while others of us battle the tendency to gain weight all our lives.

It's tempting to attribute the difference between the fat and thin among us to metabolic conditions, and I don't doubt that they play a significant role. Yet research also presents a convincing picture of an overweight population who behave differently from their slim counterparts.

I want to add here that the studies conducted on this subject usually compare visibly overweight people to normal-weight individuals. My experience has convinced me that there are many normal-weight people who think and behave like the overweight. Some people who have five pounds to lose struggle more obsessively than those with fifty. Many people who are enviably thin are that way because they are preoccupied with their diets. I'm not talking about people with serious eating disorders like anorexia nervosa. I'm referring to a wide cross section of the population who would consider themselves to be "normally neurotic."

Consequently, you don't need to be overweight to have a fat appetite.

What do I mean by a fat appetite? Here are a few examples: In one experiment, obese and non-obese volunteers arrived at a laboratory without having eaten breakfast. Their stomach contractions were recorded and they were asked if they felt hungry. The thin volunteers exhibited a close correlation between their contractions and reports of hunger. The obese showed no coincidence between the two. They had an appetite for breakfast, even if they were not physically hungry.

In another study, volunteers were fed huge roast beef sandwiches and then asked to rate flavored crackers. Those who were overweight consumed many more crackers than their similarly stuffed, non-obese counterparts.

In still another study, clocks were changed to show a 6:00 P.M. dinner time when it was actually 5:30. Obese individuals started to eat at the bogus time. Normal-weight volunteers waited until they got hungry.

The pattern is obvious. The overweight are not in tune with internal clues regarding hunger and are easily influenced by environmental circumstances. But don't be fooled into thinking that the overweight use any excuse to eat. In fact, it seems that they are far more particular about what they eat than are those of normal weight.

Studies with good-tasting and bad-tasting milk shakes and ice cream confirm that the overweight consumed much more of the good-tasting item than normal-weight subjects and much less of the bad-tasting food. The results held regardless of prior food deprivation, which reinforces the point that to the overweight, taste was more influential than hunger. Numerous studies confirm the importance of taste, esthetic appeal, environment, and other such factors to the obese.

You can see that hunger is not as influential to a fat appetite as it is to a thin one. This is a major factor to consider, because most people worry about being hungry on a diet. First of all, you won't be hungry on *The Bloomingdale's Eat Healthy Diet,* ever. But second, it's important to understand that hunger isn't really the problem.

Let me relate the findings of just one more experiment. In a study by Yale University researchers, obese and non-obese shoppers were interviewed at a New Haven supermarket. Some shoppers had eaten, others had not; those who had not were labled "deprived" for the purposes of the study.

The results of the survey revealed that obese shoppers purchased more food if they had recently eaten, and less food if they had not. Non-obese shoppers were the reverse. The researchers concluded that being deprived of food does not increase the appetite of the obese. On the contrary, the process of eating seems to trigger a greater interest in food. Normal-weight individuals, on the other hand, behave as one would expect, exhibiting more interest in food when they are physically hungry.

Therefore, although you may be able to become more sensitive to your internal physical response to hunger, the reality is that just the act of eating triggers your appetite. And you will be eating for the rest of your life. There is a silver lining to what seems like a dark cloud, however. It is wonderful to be able to love food. It is a potential source of great pleasure. Appetite Training uses your natural predisposition toward food as an asset. You will be concentrating on eating to become thin, because abstaining is clearly not a realistic long-term solution for you.

The Origins of Appetite

Even though hunger may not be the most influential aspect of appetite for the overweight, it is, of course, important. Webster's defines appetite first as "Some craving of the body." And hunger does produce a powerful craving sensation.

The first experiments on appetite were done at the turn of this century. They established the link between hunger and stomach contractions—what we think of as hunger pangs. Everyone has had the experience of these sensations, as well as the sometimes embarrassing accompanying growling noises that signal physical hunger. These sensations are helpful in reminding "thin appetites" that they need to eat. (Some people actually do forget!) For the overweight, however, hunger pangs often lead to overeating.

The Bloomingdale's Eat Healthy Diet is designed so that you never need to feel hungry. In fact, if you feel hungry, you're probably not eating enough. It isn't necessary, however, to feel full all the time, or stuffed. It's a question of balance. Letting yourself experience a degree of hunger is desirable. It can be a result of cutting down on unnecessary, reflexive eating and can also be pleasurable, enhancing your appetite and adding a sense of anticipation to a meal. But if you allow yourself to become very hungry, so that you have strong hunger pangs, you are more likely to overeat as a reaction.

It is also important to recognize that there are numerous stimuli that trigger appetite. Being in a movie can make you crave popcorn. The setting sun can make you think of dinner. Feeling disappointed can trigger a desire for ice cream. Sometimes, what you want to do is eat, and it isn't related to hunger at all.

The Stabilization phase will help you learn to handle these reflexive cravings effectively, including indulging them when that's appropriate. "It's been really important to me to know that I can 'pig out' when I feel I need to," Angie told me recently. Angie had eighty-five pounds to lose and is halfway to her goal. "You know, there are times when what I need to do is to crawl under the covers and eat. I know I'm not hungry but that doesn't necessarily help. Usually it's when I'm blue about something, and in the past I would have compounded the problem by feeling guilty because I overate. Now I've learned which foods will satisfy my emotional cravings as well as my physical ones. It's made all the difference!"

Learning which foods will satisfy you under various circumstances is part of what makes Appetite Training work. To help you become more aware of what stimulates your appetite it's useful to consider the following.

The Role of Taste and Texture

No matter how much you want to lose weight, it shouldn't be at the expense of enjoying the pleasures of food. So what are the components of the sensations that we consider to be pleasurable? You don't need scientific studies to tell you that taste is critical to your enjoyment of food, yet several studies have been conducted to confirm that fact. In one, a laboratory rat on a monotonous diet of food pellets wasn't obese, and never overate. When it was presented with a bonanza of supermarket fare, however, it acted just like we do; it gorged itself on salami, chocolate, marshmallows, and peanut butter. Eventually it turned into a very obese rat. After returning to its original diet of monotonous food pellets, it returned to its original weight as well.

Studies on humans confirm that when tempting food is involved, they behave just like laboratory rats: they overeat. And, since we know that the appetites of the overweight are more likely to be stimulated by eating delicious food, the pattern that gets you into trouble becomes obvious. The value of Appetite Training may be becoming more evident to you. After all, if you can actually change what you perceive to be delicious, you can avoid the harmful consequences of indulging your appetite.

There's a related issue that's worth mentioning here. Recently there's been a surge of low-calorie substitutes for high-calorie foods. Although these may help some people lose weight in the short run, they may perpetuate behavior that leads to overeating. A prominent doctor at Yale fears that the attempt to make low-calorie, sweet-tasting food desirable may actually stimulate appetite. This is an issue I'll be discussing again when we get into the Transition phase. For now, just bear in mind that all that diet soda and sugarless gum you consume may not be having the effect you want them to have.

The sixteenth-century French humorist François Rabelais summed it up when he said, *"L'appetit vient en mangeant"* (The appetite comes with the eating). And when you consider how we're bombarded with stimuli to tempt our salt- and sweet-sensitive tastebuds, it's easy to see how the problem escalates. Commercials come over our TVs and radios every few minutes. Print ads and posters call out to us from every available, imaginable, smooth, print-on-able surface.

Food, it seems, is available everywhere; not just at the supermarket and grocery store, but in drug stores, discount stores, even gas stations. Heaven forbid that we may be out of reach of some snack or other for even a few minutes in our normal day. And the foods being touted, and those most readily available, are not the fresh, nutritious, ideal body-building variety. Instead, they are most often the sugar-, fat-, and salt-rich snack foods that reinforce our worst appetite response and undermine the physical health of our bodies. It's no wonder we have appetites that don't respond to what's best and, in fact, most natural for our well-being.

Taste, however, is not the only element involved in temptation. There is evidence that the feel of food in our mouths may be even more important to us than the way it tastes.

A series of experiments at New York's Hunter College demonstrated that it was the oral sensations during eating that were the greater stimulus to appetite. Animals that could taste their food, but not feel it as they chewed, spent much less time eating. They seemed to totally lose interest in food.

There is human evidence that backs up those results. It's not hard to understand why the texture of food is so critical. Do you really taste the potato chips after half the bag is gone? Yet, it's a phenomenon to discover someone who can stop at half a bag. We crave the crunch. It's essential to recognize the importance of texture to appetite appeal. *The Bloomingdale's Eat Healthy Diet* is ever mindful of the fact that crunching seems to be a biological need.

Are You a Food Addict?

You don't need a great deal of scientific evidence to illustrate the dimensions of the problem. You are undoubtedly very aware of the power of your own worst cravings. Dorothy isn't alone in feeling panicked at the thought of not having what she desires close at hand. Another Workshop participant got a laugh of recognition when she said that her floor sagged into a distinct curve on the route between her TV and her refrigerator.

We are addicted to the foods we love and our habits regarding the circumstances under which we eat. What's more, there are physiological considerations that strengthen the hold of at least two of the most troublesome food addictions.

Sugar and salt are two major sources of food addictions. If you've got a sweet tooth, or are a chip or pretzel muncher, you know how hard it is to "kick the habit." The problem isn't just that you lack willpower. There is a scientific basis for the phenomenon of sweet- and salt-aholics.

As I said earlier, our tastebuds are sensitive to four varieties of taste: sweet, salty, sour, and bitter. We are especially sensitive to the last two because they warn us of harmful substances. But we need higher concentrations of sweet and salty tastes before a response can be perceived. The more sweet and salty foods we eat, the higher the sugar and salt concentration needs to be in order for us to taste those flavors. In other words, our thresholds for these tastes get higher. Physiologists call this phenomenon *adaptation*. It's easy to see why adaptation can have profound consequences, leading to behavior that is addictive. If you doubt the magnitude of the problem, consider the following.

Studies on rats reveal a fascinating relationship between alcohol abuse and sweet abuse. In one study, rats were offered a water solution and an alcohol solution. Over a period of time, the rats, not surprisingly, demonstrated a marked preference for the alcohol solution. Next, a progressively concentrated sweet solution was offered as an alternative to the alcohol. Soon, the rats began to prefer the sweet solution to the alcohol. What's incredible is that this preference occurred in rats who had had a prior affinity for alcohol.

Of course, the problem isn't limited to sugar and salt. I've learned in Eat Healthy Workshops that the basis of the other most common addictions tends to be fat. Some people are particularly attached to mayonnaise, peanut butter, cheese, olive oil, even olives. While you're dependent on your addiction, the thought of giving it up is anxiety-producing, to say the least. Once conquered, however, you'll wonder why you ever thought it was worth being fat over.

What's reassuring is that unlike giving up cigarettes or alcohol, conquering your food addictions requires no extended period of withdrawal—if it's done properly. What's more, you'll find that the process is more enjoyable than not.

Whatever your trouble spots, they'll be transitory in nature. Most often you'll feel excited as you see yourself respond in positive ways, as the weight comes off just as promised.

What's particularly interesting is that the reward of losing weight is only the beginning. The increase in energy and feelings of well-being are things that most people don't know how to anticipate. Yet you'll discover that these bonus rewards may come to mean more to you in time than your primary weight-loss goal.

3

It's Not Just Your Body, It's Your Life

Have you ever asked yourself why you want to lose weight? To be thinner. Obviously. To look better. Right. To improve your social life, or your sex life, or your confidence. How about all three? Most of us are motivated by vanity at the inception of any diet. And there's nothing wrong with that. Certainly, losing weight will help make your most vain fantasies real.

There's another powerful reason for losing weight. It's called your life. Losing weight is critical not only for the length of your life, but also for its quality. And it's not just a matter of eating less. It's what you eat less of that makes a significant contribution to lengthening and enriching your life.

Food lovers believe that, perhaps with the exception of sex, food is their greatest source of pleasure. What they don't often realize is that it is also their greatest source of pain. Not just psychic and emotional pain, but also the physical pain that accompanies a body that isn't fueled to operate properly.

Meet the Caretaker of Your Body—You

Your enjoyment in life is directly linked to the condition of your body. You can experience life only through your body, so it makes sense that you're dependent upon it for your pleasures. What's sad is that most of us live lives that are greatly restricted because of our bodies. We're so used to the way we feel that we don't even notice what we're missing.

You probably think it feels great at the end of the day when you can sit down and "take a load off your feet." You may be so accustomed to the aches and pains with which you live that you consider a good day one in which you're not hurting. It's a negative approach to health. There's an old saying that goes, "If you think you're miserable, you should put on a tight shoe. You'll be so thrilled to take it off, you'll forget whatever it was that was troubling you." It's a life-limiting approach to your body.

I maintain that you don't even remember what it feels like to feel great. What's more, you might feel vaguely uncomfortable with the whole notion of doing something about it. We're often tempted to hold onto our physical complaints (overweight being just one of them) as our built-in excuse for the things we don't want to do in life.

What you need to consider is the price you pay for your neglect. After all, you only live once. This isn't a dress rehearsal. This is your life—and your body. You don't get to trade it in for a new model when it wears out. You're only going to get to live this life with this body. Now, it's up to you to determine the quality of both!

It's not your body's fault, by the way. You may hate your body for the extra rolls of fat it carries around. You may feel cheated because you're not the physical type you wish you were. You may envy others whom you believe can eat more than you can, or whom you imagine enjoy exercise more than you do. Remember, I've admitted that life isn't fair.

Now you have to admit that most of the body beautifuls you see around you didn't happen by accident. People in peak physical shape work at it. So, my advice to you is stop fighting it. Join it!

A New Look at Nutrition

Unless you've been living under a rock, you know that the typical American diet (high fat, low complex carbohydrate, high simple carbohydrate) has been linked to the nation's top killers: heart disease, atherosclerosis, hypertension, stroke, diabetes, and certain cancers. Genetics, environment, and untold other factors also play a role, but diet is a factor we can learn to control with Effective Appetite Training. In addition, obesity in itself is a main risk factor associated with adult-onset diabetes, hypertension, and heart disease. Your "excess baggage" may also be causing orthopedic problems —such as nagging backaches.

The good news is that an improved diet can offer protections from the devastating effects of ill health. The question many people have today is, "What constitutes a healthy diet?" It's genuinely confusing, since the latest recommendations contradict the dogma on which most of us were reared.

We all know that food is composed of fat, carbohydrate, and protein, and that all three play a role in a proper diet. Recent evidence, however, indicates that the balance of these three dietary components is the problem with our current diet. What's needed to prevent disease and promote good health and slender, sexy bodies is a major turnaround in our assumptions about what's good for us.

Most Americans get almost half their calories from fat; estimates range from 40 to 50 percent. That figure needs to come way down. The most conservative estimates say that our maximum fat intake should not exceed 30 percent of daily calories. Many respected medical and scientific authorities put the desirable range of fat calories at 10 to 15 percent of an optimum diet. Because our primary goal is weight loss, and no one suggests that a low-fat diet is in any way harmful, I recommend aiming for the lower fat intake. This means you need to increase your consumption of either protein or carbohydrate to make up the difference.

The surprise for many is that it's the carbohydrate you want to increase, not the protein. To understand why, let's look at each dietary component separately.

FAT

There's no way around it: Fat is the enemy. Whether it's in the form of saturated fat, which is solid at room temperature (and which is the cholesterol-carrying kind), or unsaturated fat, which is liquid, fat is the most concentrated form of food energy you can eat. "Isn't that good?" you might wonder. After all, energy is good, right? Not when it's used to describe food! Energy is synonymous with calories. Fat contains nine calories per gram versus only four calories per gram for carbohydrate and protein. In other words, it doesn't take much fat to make you gain weight. For example, one tablespoon of butter has the same number of calories as a medium baked potato.

And fat is ubiquitous. It's in just about everything you love: butter, margarine, oils of all kinds, mayonnaise, sour cream, cream cheese, all cheese for that matter, cream, whole milk, cakes, cookies, most candy, nuts, seeds, anything containing shortening, meat, chicken, even fish. Sometimes you can see the fat, sometimes you can't. Just know that the steak you think is so good for you may calorically be 70 percent fat.

It's worthwhile to review the tables beginning on page 181 to become familiar with the fat content of various foods. For example, notice what happens to a potato, which contains no fat, when you eat it as hash browns (page 209); or notice that nuts and seeds (page 204), which you might have considered "healthy" because of their protein content, also contain an unhealthy quantity of fat—and consequently calories.

We need fat in our bodies to metabolize certain vitamins, to cushion our vital organs, and to provide insulation, which helps us maintain a constant body temperature, winter and summer. We don't need a lot of fat, however; certainly nowhere near the amount most of us carry around. And we don't have to ingest much dietary fat to get the benefits we need. Our bodies, efficient machines that they are, convert all excess calories to fat, no matter what the source. In fact, you undoubtedly will get more fat than you "need" on even the most restricted diets, as long as you're eating grains, fish, chicken, and vegetables. In addition, even though you will learn how to order in restaurants to avoid high-fat foods, chances are you will be getting unanticipated fats in the foods you don't prepare yourself.

Fat and Disease Beyond the fattening qualities of fat, there are the health dangers. In 1956, when the U.S. Department of Agriculture (USDA) first established the four basic food groups—dairy, meat, fruits and vegetables, and breads and cereals—it was assumed that eating from all four groups would ensure a healthy diet. By the early 1960s, however, researchers were reporting findings that indicated a link between dairy products and meat—both of which contain a high percentage of fat—and degenerative diseases, such as heart disease, stroke, hypertension, and obesity.

In 1977, the Senate Select Committee on Nutrition and Human Needs published a far-reaching report that was the culmination of almost ten years of investigation. It found the evidence linking diet to disease overwhelming, and recommended that everyone cut consumption of fat, cholesterol, sugar, and salt to help combat disease.

About a year later, the findings of the thirty-year Framingham heart study were published. This exhaustive, landmark study involved more than five thousand adults whose diets were scrutinized over the entire thirty-year period. The study revealed strong evidence of a prevalence of coronary heart disease in people who had high levels of blood cholesterol, high blood pressure, and a history of cigarette smoking. Recent updates to the Framingham study have caused those reviewing the data to state that the three factors just mentioned are not just "associated risk factors," but actually cause heart disease. Dr. William P. Castelli, the medical director of the Framingham study, stated rather dramatically that "the striking, overriding fact is that the first sign of underlying coronary heart disease all too often is death, and very frequently sudden death, before any effective therapeutic measures can be administered. Obviously then, the only answer to conquering this disease is effective primary prevention." Effective primary prevention begins with revising your diet to reduce your intake of fat and salt and, if you haven't already done so, stopping smoking.

More recently, fat has been linked to another dreaded killer, cancer. In 1982, the Committee on Diet, Nutrition and Cancer of the National Research Council issued a report that offered evidence linking a high-fat diet to cancers of the colon and breast and possibly to cancers of the prostate and ovaries.

It's quite a responsibility when you stop and think about it. You can actually alter the odds of your contracting heart disease or cancer, or suffering a debilitating or deadly stroke.

Note: Before we leave the subject of fat, just a clarifying word about cholesterol. Cholesterol is not fat, although it is usually mentioned along with fat. Cholesterol is actually a sterol and contains no calories. It is produced naturally in the liver and is contained in meat, eggs, and dairy foods. High cholesterol levels are an indication of an increased risk of heart disease, atherosclerosis, and stroke. Remember, however, that cholesterol isn't the only risk factor. Excess unsaturated fats are also harmful (and as fattening as saturated fats).

PROTEIN

All living things depend on protein and require it in order to grow. Every cell in your body contains it. Protein is a lifelong necessity for maintaining a healthy body. No question. The problem with protein comes from a widespread misconception that we need a lot of it. People worry about whether or not they're getting "enough" protein.

I can put your mind at rest. You are getting enough protein. Believe me. You're probably getting much, much more than you need or, in fact, than is good for you. All you "need," day to day, is to replace the small amounts that are lost in the process of life. The RDA (Recommended Daily Allowance) for protein is only forty-four grams per day for the average woman and fifty-six grams per day for the average man. As a safety factor, the RDA is computed to be substantially higher than the average individual requirements. Low-fat dairy products, grains, and many vegetables contain generous amounts of protein. So you need only one serving (three to four ounces each) of legumes, fish, poultry, or lean meat a day to supply the rest.

What's more, it's now known that you can be getting too much protein. Your body will take what it needs and store the rest, as fat, for future use. Since you already have plenty of stored fat, and you probably eat protein every day, excessive amounts of protein will serve only to contribute to increasing your risk of gout or an enlarged liver. It also leads to calcium loss (of particular importance to women) because the process of digesting protein depletes the body of minerals. In animals, excess protein has also been linked to an inflammation of the kidneys.

The final thing you need to know about protein is that the most common sources of it are meat and dairy foods. Both, as you well know, contain high levels of fat (sometimes, as in the case of butter, as much as 85 percent). So if you're someone who believes you need a lot of protein, you need to recognize that the cost of clinging to that myth is fattening!

CARBOHYDRATE

Now for the good news. Carbohydrate, which most dieters have routinely avoided, is the mainstay of the new nutrition. During the past fifty years, Americans have dramatically reduced their consumption of complex carbohydrates. We now need to reverse that trend.

The secret to understanding how to use carbohydrate to lose weight and to prevent disease is in the difference between the two forms in which it is found: simple and complex. Simple carbohydrates are sugars, which contain minimal nutrients. Complex carbohydrates are starches—such as whole-wheat and whole-grain breads and cereals, vegetables, legumes, fruit, brown rice, millet, barley, oats, and whole-wheat pasta—which are rich in vitamins, minerals, and protein.

So it's complex carbohydrates that you need to include in your diet. And many of the foods you've denied yourself when you've dieted in the past are the ones you will be eating now: bread, pasta, rice, and potatoes, for example. It's most important that you look for breads, cereals, and pasta that have not been highly processed, because whole grains contain the most food value.

Besides providing a relatively low-calorie source of nutrients, there's another important bonus you get from complex carbohydrates: fiber. Fiber is what remains of complex carbohydrate foods after digestion. The fiber itself contains no nutrients, but provides bulk, which absorbs water to make you feel full. Constipation is a major problem for millions of Americans and the laxative effect of fiber helps prevent it. In addition, it is believed that a high-fiber diet contributes to preventing colon and rectal cancers, hemorrhoids, gallstones, hiatus hernias, diverticulosis, arteriosclerosis, and other prevalent conditions.

For our purposes, however, the greatest benefit of complex carbohydrates is as a boon to dieters. Fresh vegetables, fruits, and grains provide delicious and filling fare from which to build an endless variety of meals. *The Bloomingdale's Eat Healthy Diet* will teach you how to use complex carbohydrates easily as the focus of your meals. You'll find you feel full longer due to the high fiber content of the diet. And, besides losing weight, you'll know that you may be reversing the consequences of years of mistreating your body. The rewards will be measured not only in a thinner waistline, but also in the possibility of added years of health and vitality.

FORGET THE SUGAR, DON'T PASS THE SALT

You already know what you're about to read. You know how bad salt and sugar are for you. You've read that salt is a major contributor to hypertension. You know that sugar supplies only empty calories. But have you given them up? Probably not.

Americans get as much as 25 percent of their daily calories from refined sugar alone. This simple carbohydrate is frequently the source of complex patterns of overeating. Because it metabolizes so quickly in the body, it isn't satisfying. The familiar pattern is to feel a quick "up" after eating sugar, and then a sensation of sinking, once your glucose level plunges. The worst part is that eating sugar usually stimulates your appetite for more. It is also a major cause of dental worries, so you would be wise to cut it out even if you didn't want to lose a pound. In addition, there is evidence that complex carbohydrates help prevent heart disease. Too many people consume simple rather than complex carbohydrates, and therefore lose out on important health benefits. But for anyone who is overweight, sugar should be thought of as a poison.

Unfortunately, sugar is present in just about everything. So is salt. I'm mentioning these two no-no's together because if a prepared or processed food doesn't contain one, it's bound to contain the other. Many canned, frozen, and packaged foods contain both. It's not just the salt that comes out of the shaker, or the sugar from the sugar bowl, that you need to eliminate. You're getting added salt or sugar in everything from canned tomatoes to breakfast cereal.

Consequently, I have placed a heavy emphasis on fresh foods in all phases of *The Bloomingdale's Eat Healthy Diet*. Both sugar and salt do occur naturally in fresh produce, but in amounts most of us can easily tolerate. Some of the recipes in Chapter 8 call for ingredients that contain some sugar and salt. Again, these are used in such small amounts that they're inconsequential—if you're not also ingesting the dangerous duo from other sources.

Note: If you have high blood pressure you'll need to watch the salt content of some of the recipes suggested. Although you will be cutting way down on your salt intake relative to your current diet, some recipes call for ingredients that contain more salt than is desirable for someone with hypertension. I point them out in the recipe chapter and recommend substitutions, but it's wise to keep it in mind, since we all have a tendency to skip around when we read recipes, and you might miss the hints if you're not looking for them.

Incidentally, if you don't have a complicating medical condition, it isn't necessary to be overly vigilant regarding salt. Some salt is required for normal physiological functions. The Recommended Daily Allowance for sodium is 1,100 to 3,300 milligrams for adults. One teaspoon of salt has 2,000 milligrams of sodium.

Defying a Sedentary Lifestyle

To talk about losing weight, getting in shape, and protecting your body against unnecessary disease without including exercise would be a gross disservice. Our sedentary lifestyle plays a major role in increasing the risk of cardiovascular illness, as well as compounding the problem of obesity.

Not long ago, the majority of Americans gave little thought to exercise. Even in the early 1970s, when jogging replaced dropping out as the national obsession, it was considered a phenomenon for "fitness nuts." Today, however, there are ninety million of us who exercise regularly, and our ranks are swelling daily.

It's no wonder when you add up the benefits of vigorous exercise. To get the most from an exercise program, it should be aerobic in nature, that is, one that works your heart muscle more rigorously than the stretching and bending of simple calisthenics.

Aerobic exercise requires oxygen for prolonged periods. Consequently, your body actually produces new blood vessels to help carry the increased oxygen to your heart. This, in turn, benefits your entire circulatory system. In addition, aerobic exercise increases the capacity of your lungs, which some studies have associated with greater longevity. It also strengthens your heart muscle and lowers cholesterol levels. And, while exercising, your brain releases endorphins, which act as a natural tranquilizer. So regular aerobic exercise reduces stress and elevates your mood.

If all of the above isn't enough to send you in search of jogging shoes, consider the positive effects of exercise on weight loss. If you pair your exercise with a diet, your body will have to go into its fat reserves to get the additional energy required to keep your heart pumping and your blood circulating. I want to repeat that a forty-five-minute workout will burn off anywhere from 200 to 400 calories, or more if you make it really strenuous. Recent studies show that you will continue to burn calories at a higher rate for as long as twenty-four hours after an aerobic workout, so the benefits may continue to work, even when you're not working out.

Of course, you won't just be burning calories and aiding your heart, lungs, and circulatory system; you'll also be toning your muscles. You'll look thinner as you build muscles because muscle tissue takes up less space than fat. The fact is that long-term studies of formerly overweight people show that those who integrate exercise into their daily lives have an easier time maintaining their weight loss. There's little doubt why.

Finding the Right Exercise Program for You

The thing about exercise is that it doesn't work if all you do is think about it. You actually have to get out there and sweat if you want to reap the benefits. And, as I said, most overweight people are particularly reluctant to get active. This is one of those times when you have to push yourself. You can't believe how great you'll feel until you've been at it for a few weeks. And even after you're convinced that it's as terrific for body and soul as everyone claims, you'll still have to press yourself to keep at it when you're feeling low or tired, or when it's raining.

It's important to approach an exercise program in a methodical way. If you're very overweight, have been sedentary for years, or have any potentially complicating physical condition, you should check with your doctor before you begin. In fact, it's wise to get a checkup before beginning an exercise program regardless of your current condition.

The key to arriving at the proper level of activity for yourself is to monitor your optimum exercise heart rate. To compute this number, first subtract your age from the number 220. This will give you your age-adjusted maximum heart rate per minute. It is recommended that people under fifty years of age exercise at a rate of 80 percent of their age-adjusted maximum; those over fifty at 75 percent; those over sixty at 70 percent. So, if you're forty, your optimum heart rate during aerobic exercise is twenty-four beats per ten seconds. To verify your rate of exertion as you exercise, you should stop periodically and take your pulse. There are two easy places to check your pulse. The first is on your wrist, just beneath your thumb. Use the third and fourth fingers of one hand to apply light pressure on the wrist of the other. The other easy pulse point to find is just to the side of your Adam's apple. Again, use the same two fingers to press *lightly* against your neck. Use the second hand on a watch or clock to gauge ten seconds while you count your pulse beats.

	220	220	220
Age	− 40	− 55	− 65
Age-adjusted maximum heart rate per minute	180	165	155
	× .80	× .75	× .70
Optimum heart rate per minute for exercise	144	124	109
	÷ 6	÷ 6	÷ 6
Ten-second count	24	21	18

If all this sounds confusing to you, slow down and read the above paragraphs again. It's really very easy—and it's very important. Overexertion is potentially dangerous. What you want to do is aim for a program that will work your heart at its optimum rate for an extended period of time. Your goal should be forty-five to sixty minutes, four to six days a week. You won't be working at your optimum rate for the full forty-five or sixty minutes, but it's desirable to build up endurance. Take your time working up to your time goal.

You should exercise a minimum of four days a week. Although many experts agree that you can derive the benefits from aerobic exercise if you do it three days a week, my experience has shown me that those who exercise more often tend to love exercising. At the three-times-a-week level, there's a tendency to think of it as a chore. At the five-times-a-week level, it becomes a way of life—something to look forward to. I recommend that you build up to four to six days a week and you'll find yourself addicted in no time. And this is one addiction that's good for you! The Transition phase includes a walking program to get you started. Don't rush yourself. You'll know when you feel ready to increase.

What activity is best for you? Here's a brief rundown on several popular options. You'll see that there is a wide range of choices that require little equipment or special expertise. Any of these will give you the workout you need:

Walking. Brisk walking is an ideal way to begin exercising. Many couples walk together before dinner. It sure beats having a drink to unwind, and it will curb your appetite and undoubtedly improve your relationship! Be sure to wear comfortable shoes and to swing your arms freely. Strolling will not give your heart the workout it needs. Take your pulse every five minutes or so in the beginning, until you reach your optimum level. Once your walking program is established, you may find you need to step up your pace, or move on to a different activity to keep your heart rate up.

Jogging. It's easy to get addicted to jogging. All you need is a good pair of running shoes and you're in business. It's easier on your body to jog on a dirt road or a grass surface. Pavement is fine, however, as long as your shoes are well cushioned. The key is to start very slowly, barely faster than a walk. If your pulse rate gets too high, slow down but don't stop moving. A portable cassette player with a headset, or a friend to jog with, will help make the time fly by.

Swimming. Swimming is one of the most popular ways to exercise, but it's one option that does require some expertise because you'll get a better workout if you have a strong stroke. It's well worth taking classes at your local Y or swim club. This will improve your stroke as well as motivate you to attend on a regular basis. Swimming is considered an ideal form of overall body conditioning. You'll need a long pool or a natural body of water to make it aerobically effective. If you have to stop frequently to turn, you'll cut down on the benefits. If you have difficulty getting your heart rate up while you swim, alternate it with another activity.

Bicycling. To make bicycling your primary form of exercise, you need to have the right kind of terrain. If your area is too hilly, or if you live in a city where there are lots of traffic lights, you may have a problem. To reap the benefits, you'll need relatively flat, open spaces. Bicycling isn't as jarring as many other forms of aerobic activity and may be ideal if you have problems with your knees or ankles. Beware of overdoing it when you begin. Your heart rate may be fine, but your leg muscles might complain if you're too ambitious at first.

Stationary Bicycling. This requires a special piece of equipment—either an indoor trainer stand for your regular bicycle or an exercise bicycle—but it's well worth it. Once you get in the habit, exercising on a stationary bicycle is very easy to work into your day. Lots of people enjoy a stationary bike because they can watch TV while they work their heart muscles. If you like a set routine, this may be the way to go.

Jumping Rope. Jumping rope is great if you're in shape and want to augment another form of exercise. It will get your heart rate up quickly and give you an excellent aerobic workout in a short period of time. Still, endurance is important and it's difficult not to exceed your optimum exercise heart rate unless you're vigilant. Begin very cautiously: Check your pulse every minute or two. It's worth practicing jumping rope because it's so easy to do it anywhere, anytime, rain or shine. Begin by using an alternate step. Jumping with both feet together is more strenuous and more jarring to your body. Well-cushioned tennis shoes are ideal footwear.

Aerobic Dancing/Exercise Class   Join a class, buy a tape, or choose your favorite upbeat music and go it alone. Whichever route you take, aerobic exercise or dancing is great fun. If you choose dancing, don't worry about steps or "doing it right." Just let yourself feel the beat and keep up with it. Tennis shoes are better than running shoes for aerobic dancing, since they are designed to move sideways, as well as forward and back.

How to Begin

Choose one option and commit yourself to it for a minimum of four days a week. Don't shy away from classes. Working out with others will make it more fun. I recommend that you concentrate on one activity because I believe it reinforces your resolve to make it a consistent habit. If you switch off too much, especially at first, it becomes hard to settle into a routine.

Be certain to warm up before you begin. Stretch slowly, first by extending your arms over your head, and then swinging them from side to side. You can stretch out your calf muscles easily by sitting on the floor, extending your legs in front of you, bending at the waist, and reaching for your toes with your hands. Alternately point and flex your toes for a few counts. When you complete your exercise for the day, be sure to take a few moments to cool down. Don't stop abruptly. Walk around slowly for several minutes. Stretch your arm and leg muscles again. A good warm-up and cooldown will help prevent aching muscles later on.

Don't try to make up for a sedentary past too quickly. Build up slowly. Let your heart rate be your guide. The most important thing is to be consistent. Make exercise a priority; your body will say "thank you."

Boundless Energy—Can This Be You?

The result of the new nutrition and an active exercise program is an increased energy for living that will amaze you. You can't even imagine how different you'll feel.

Most of us don't really believe that we are what we eat, or we wouldn't dream of eating the way we do. In the past, you probably never had the benefit of a well-orchestrated program to help you convert to ideal habits. With *The Bloomingdale's Eat Healthy Diet*, feeling terrific is a by-product of fast weight loss. Still, the balance in the diet you'll be eating is ideal for realizing the benefits of the most advanced nutritional thinking. And what you'll discover is that, believe it or not, you are what you eat.

It's tempting to let yourself off the hook with the thought that this much sugar won't matter, or that this ice cream cone won't make a difference, when you consider all the ice cream you've eaten, or that missing exercise today can't hurt, or that two days of exercise are better than none. It all matters. Every mouthful. Every day of exercise. If you want to look like your ideal body image, every day counts. If you want to wake up feeling sensational, instead of barely alive, every day counts. If you want to live a long and healthy life, every day counts. And if you don't want to look and feel sensational, and live to a ripe old age, what do you want?

4

The Transition Phase

The best place to start the Transition phase is in front of a full-length mirror—with the lights on. Many people have the amazing ability to see only what they need to see when they look in a mirror. You can check if that shirt goes with this jacket, or if your hair is combed. But it's easy to let your eyes glaze over and take in only the overall impression, rather than concentrate on the specific reality of *you*.

What I want you to do is really look at yourself. It is best to do this naked, but if that's hard for you, do it fully dressed. Really examine yourself and let yourself feel all the feelings that surface as you do. Some of them may be very negative, others positive. Remember, however, that you are looking at a you that is about to be past tense.

You used to be that person in the mirror. What will happen in Transition is that you will be passing into a whole new phase in your life, as well as your diet. You need to get a clear picture of who you are going to be to make that passage successful.

Creating an Ideal Body Image

Creating an ideal body image is like taking a snapshot of your future. It's the beginning of the whole Appetite Training process that will make a thin you a reality. What you're going to do is to create an image of the body you want to have, and concentrate on craving it.

Start by really wanting a better body. Begin by letting yourself imagine how different life would be if you loved looking at yourself in the mirror. Imagine going out of your way to pass a mirror, and then turning sideways so you would be sure to admire your body in profile. No protruding stomach; no spreading hips.

Let yourself get more specific. Create a very real picture of your perfect dream body. Are you naked or dressed? Are you in front of a mirror or do you see yourself jogging around a track? What are you wearing? Get a very clear single image. Make sure it's you in the fantasy, and not some other person you'd like to look like. But don't limit yourself by your concept of reality. *The Bloomingdale's Eat Healthy Diet* will blow the lid off your current perception of what's possible for you. So create an ideal image that exceeds what you believe is possible, as long as you are clearly the star of it.

Be sure to include how you feel in the image. Think about those times in your life when you've felt extremely energetic, positive, and in control, and use that memory to contribute to your image. A high energy level is a critical aspect of anyone's ideal body image.

Fix your complete ideal body image firmly in your mind. Pretend it's a snapshot of the future that you can pull out to look at whenever you choose. Make certain it's real for you. You can embellish your image and expand upon it. But have a snapshot version that you can refer to easily. You must make a thin, positive you a reality for yourself. You have to know that you will look like your snapshot. You have to want all the wonderful things in your life that will come from achieving this new image you have created for yourself. I want you to crave your new body.

Participants in Eat Healthy Workshops have reported a wide range of experiences when they create their ideal body images in the first session. Some form their image immediately, as soon as I begin to talk about it. Others, like Rebecca, have a hard time.

"You know," Rebecca confided to her group the night it first met, "I've never been thin. Never. I can't imagine what to picture. In my fantasies, I look like Linda Evans, not like a thin me." Rebecca formed her image by imagining herself playing tennis, something she'd always wanted to do, but never had the confidence to try. She began by picturing her 5'3" frame weighing 115 pounds, instead of the 185 it did on that night. She cut her hair for her ideal image because she knew she wouldn't have to hide her "chipmunk cheeks" any longer. And then she put on sunglasses to help her see a face she couldn't imagine too easily. There she was, in her tennis whites, her new haircut, a bit sweaty from winning her match, as she put on her sunglasses, striding off the court. "It's like a home movie for me," she said, amazed at how real it was becoming. My only advice was to pick one frame from her movie to act as her snapshot.

Other ideal body images have run the gamut from modeling swim suits to running in a marathon. Lots of people use clothes that no longer fit them as an important element in their image. If I had to generalize, though, I'd say "great fitting jeans" is the article of clothing most often mentioned as wardrobe.

Whatever your own ideal body image is, make certain that it is really vivid before you continue. It's going to become more real for you than that old image you just said goodbye to in the mirror.

How Transition Works

You and your ideal body image are about to embark on the most profound experience you have had with food since you left mother's milk behind. You are going to reenter the world of food and eating. What the Transition phase does is create new longings; actual cravings for foods that are genuine rewards. It cleans out your system in a carefully structured manner, so that you can taste food again, or perhaps for the very first time. You will discover what it is to experience truly what you're eating. Within the first few days, you'll begin to savor flavors you can't even distinguish now.

The ten-day program works in four distinct ways to help you lose the maximum amount of weight, safely, while you are creating new cravings and learning to appreciate food in a whole new way.

First, it makes you feel as if your system has been cleansed and has been given an opportunity to return to its own natural equilibrium.

Second, this cleansing phase provides a quick weight loss that gets your diet off to an exciting start.

Third, the diet is structured to reintroduce you to foods in a way that enables you to appreciate flavor and texture as never before. By the time you are reintroduced to the sweet pleasures of a dessert, the fruit you'll be eating will taste more welcome and delicious than a bowl of your favorite ice cream would today. The same is true for healthy complex carbohydrates like brown rice and whole-grain bread, which will taste better than their more refined counterparts.

Fourth, the diet provides the basis for a long-term shift in how you relate to food, so that you are reawakened to the inherent pleasure of it while you break old, destructive (and fattening) food addictions. The result is that you not only take off hard-to-lose pounds, but also keep them off!

The ten-day plan begins with a three-day cleansing phase

during which you eat only vegetables. The other food groups are introduced one by one during the remaining week. Grains are added on the fourth day. Poultry and fish, dairy and fruit follow.

You may be wondering how all of the Transition days can be nutritionally adequate. Won't the days before Day 5 (where fish and poultry are added) be deficient in protein? The answer to this is both yes and no.

If you look at the analysis of sample menus for Transition Days 1 through 4, you'll notice that these days do provide protein. This is because vegetables do have protein. The RDA for women is only 44 grams of protein per day. The first three Transition all-vegetable days, as indicated on the prototype menus, provide you with slightly less than this. Men have a somewhat higher protein requirement (55 grams day). They can get more protein by adding another cup or so of vegetables to Transition Days 1 through 4. After Transition Day 4 you will receive protein in excess of the RDA for men and women. It is also important to note that the RDA for protein is estimated to exceed the requirement of most persons. Therefore, intakes below the RDA are not necessarily inadequate.

It is true that a solely vegetable diet (without legumes and grains) will not provide you with complete proteins (ones that provide you with all the protein building blocks your body cannot manufacture), but by eating a great variety of vegetables you are more likely to obtain all the nutrients you need. Remember, you are training your appetite. To obtain the full benefit of this process you might initially tip the protein scale a bit. Transition is also for such a short period of time that it should not be harmful to any persons in good health.

In addition, the three-day all-vegetable phase of Transition is a period needed to quickly purge you of your old, detrimental eating habits. It allows you to enjoy trying new vegetables of delicious and different colors, shapes, textures, and tastes!

Before we get into the specifics of the ten-day plan, it's helpful to set your weight-loss goals. Setting concrete goals encourages you to achieve them. If you're not specific, it's easier to be fuzzy about your commitment. When you know exactly where you're aiming, it makes it easier to hit the mark.

Setting Your Goals

I want you to set two weight-loss goals: one for the Transition phase itself, the other for your Ideal Body Image. Each goal needs a specific timetable.

For the Transition phase, you know that you're dealing with a ten-day time span. Most people take off anywhere from five to twelve pounds during this phase. If you have less than fifteen pounds to lose, or you have just lost weight, you will probably end up at the lower end of the range. If you have more weight to lose and haven't lost any recently, you should aim at the high end. In my experience, by the way, men lose faster than women. There have been people who have lost more than twelve pounds and some fewer than five, but they are the exceptions. I recommend that you be optimistic in setting your goal. Use the parameters I've laid out and then "go for it." If you set a slightly high goal for yourself, you'll be that much more vigilant and less likely to take advantage of the unlimited food you are allowed to eat.

Now, commit to your goal. Use a pencil so that if you want to go through Transition again, you can remake it.

TRANSITION WEIGHT-LOSS GOAL: _____
TIME PERIOD: <u>10 DAYS</u>

Your Ideal Body Image goal will take more thought. I've noticed in Eat Healthy Workshops that people with a great deal of weight to lose usually underestimate their goal. Conversely, those with ten extra pounds or so usually overestimate and set themselves an unrealistically high target. You can always refine your goal as you go along.

It's important to recognize that losing weight happens in stages. Periodically, your body will need to adjust to its new weight and you will hit a plateau. It's part of the process. So you need to figure that time into your calculations. It's also important that you not set too demanding a timetable. A slower weight loss will be much easier to maintain, and much healthier to achieve. If you're faithful to the program, you will probably double your Transition loss within the first month. After that, you will begin to lose more slowly, but still steadily. If you do plateau for an extended period, you can speed yourself through it by going on Transition again.

In general, if you have a lot of weight to lose, I want you to double the time you think you need to take it all off. Although this may sound contrary to the advice I gave in setting your goal for Transition, it's not. Transition is designed for quick weight loss. Stabilization is designed for permanent weight loss. The techniques required to achieve the results are different. Face it, if you lost half your weight in a given time period, and it stayed off, you'd be thrilled. If you make life too strictly regimented, for too long a period of time, you're setting yourself up for the "all-or-nothing" kind of thinking that leads to failure. So though it's perfectly possible to take off fifty pounds in six months, you'd be much wiser to allow yourself a full year. It's likely that the weight will come off sooner than the full year, but you'll be much more relaxed and committed if you allow yourself a reasonably achievable goal.

Realizing that this is your best guess, and that it's okay to revise it as you go along, set your goal now.

IDEAL BODY IMAGE GOAL WEIGHT: _____
TIME PERIOD: _____

As you read through the rest of this chapter, keep in mind that the more closely you adhere to the program, the faster you'll lose weight. For some people, following the rules is the hardest part of the diet. I've learned in the Workshop that people fall into two groups when it comes to following rules. One group I call the "rebels." They're the ones who consider a "One Way" traffic sign a challenge. The other group loves rules. Nothing makes them happier than clear-cut boundaries and directions. Recognize that if you're a member of the first group, all rules are irritating to you—not just these. And it's important to follow these exactly because that's the way the program works best. If you're a member of the second group, you'll love Transition and may experience more difficulty adjusting to the freedom permitted in Stabilization. Remember that in either case *you should never be hungry.* It's critical to understand that. The success of Transition is dependent upon your feelings of satisfaction. Whenever you feel hungry, you should eat. No matter how many vegetables you eat, it would be very difficult to eat as many calories as you get from your favorite dessert!

To fully understand how the diet works, first read the following rules very carefully. Then study the suggested prototype menus for all ten days (pages 56–66). Notice the summary provided in "Ten Days at a Glance" (pages 69–73), and the convenient shorthand version (page 74). Finally, read through the "Permissible Exchanges" list thoroughly (pages 75–79). You'll see that I've given you suggested menus for each of the ten days of Transition but that you don't have to follow them exactly. You can make substitutions from the "Permissible Exchanges" list whenever you choose to do so. You can even switch dinner for lunch. As long as you follow all twelve rules and eat the *number* of servings from each food group permitted each day, the "Permissible Exchanges" allow you to be as flexible as you desire.

Basic Rules of the Transition Phase

1. **Follow the recommended daily food plans exactly.**
Do not eat from a food group until it is permitted or vary the
number of servings per day from a permitted food group.
You will find that the number of servings is inconsistent
day-to-day, so you do need to follow the daily food plans very
carefully. You can check the "Ten Days at a Glance" chart
on page 74 for easy reference.

You may make substitutions from within each food group.
This is fully explained in the "Permissible Exchanges" list
(pages 75–80).

2. **Drink at least six to eight eight-ounce glasses of
water each day, without fail!** Tap water and carbonated
water are both fine. I don't mean liquids (such as coffee or
tea). I mean water—plain water. This is easy to forget as you
go through the day, and it's most important to the success of
Transition. If you have trouble drinking plain water, you can
squeeze fresh lemon juice into it.

3. **During the cleansing phase—Days 1, 2, and 3—and
through Day 8, you will be permitted two tablespoons
(six teaspoons) of plain, low-fat yogurt and half an apple
per day.** Here's where following the rules can really add
to your experience. Eating only half the apple is very important. You should choose a large apple rather than eat a whole
small one. It can be a cathartic experience to wrap half of
something and put it away for another time. You will also be
surprised at how satisfying half an apple can be. You can
use your allotted yogurt and apple in recipes (as indicated)
or as a snack. You may not substitute other fruit or dairy for
your yogurt and apple allotment. Note that starting with
Day 6, you can have up to eight ounces of Priority Dairy
products (page 77) as a snack if you don't eat them at mealtime.

4. **There is no restriction on the use of spices, herbs,**

vinegar, lemon juice, coffee (decaffeinated is preferred), tea, herbal tea, or seltzer. A note about caffeine and Transition: In general, caffeine consumption is not thought of as healthful. It is thought to contribute to birth defects, heart attacks, arrhythmias, hypertension, anxiety, fibrocystic breast disease, and it stimulates acid secretion in the stomach, which may initiate or aggravate ulcers. It is also the biggest troublemaker for people on Transition. It's a potent stimulant that may cause irritability on the diet.

I have rarely had a complaint from a non-coffee drinker about irritability. The "Catch-22" of it is that when you give up caffeine, you generally experience fatigue and sometimes a headache. If you're on Transition, you're bound to attribute these reactions to the diet. Most often, it's not the diet. You might feel a bit light-headed for brief periods of time, sometimes on the second or third day. But it's usually a very mild reaction (see "Potential Problems and Pitfalls," page 66). If you feel tired or headachy you can counteract these reactions with a staged withdrawal. Brew a half coffee/half decaffeinated drink in the beginning, slowly increasing the proportion of decaffeinated to coffee. It's well worth being tired for a few days, or having a mild headache, to rid yourself of such a potentially harmful habit.

5. Except for the seasonings and liquids already mentioned, no others are permitted, unless specifically indicated on a daily food plan. No oil, butter, margarine, sugar, baked goods, or alcohol are permitted. *Diet soda and artificial sweeteners are not allowed, because they reinforce a desire for sugar.* This is very important. For some people this is the toughest part of the program, and it is absolutely essential. Artificial sweetener in your coffee in the morning starts your day with a "sweet fix." As suggested in Chapter 2, just because artificial sweeteners contain no calories doesn't mean they don't create cravings for foods that do. There has also been much debate in the past few years over the potential harmful effects of artificial sweeteners. In addition, no fruit or

vegetable juices are allowed, because they give you calories without the satisfaction and benefits of fiber. Review the "Not Permitted" list on pages 79–80 carefully.

6. **Vegetables on the "Unlimited" list (page 75) are permitted in quantity and may be eaten, raw or cooked, at any time as a snack.** It is wise to exercise discretion, since eating exceedingly large quantities of anything is undesirable. Still, during Transition it is important not to be hungry, so feel free to indulge in vegetable snacks whenever you have the urge to eat.

7. **Unless otherwise noted, broiling, boiling, steaming, baking without oil or butter, and water sautéing (page 140) are the only acceptable cooking methods.**

8. **Always eat your grain and animal protein selections at mealtime, or during the day.** Do not "save" food for night eating. The only foods permitted after dinner are your half-apple snack (or one fruit after Day 9), vegetables, and unused Priority Dairy exchanges (after Day 6).

9. **If you go off the program at any time during the ten-day period, return with an all-vegetable day before continuing where you left off.** It's most important that you not use this rule as permission to go off the diet. It's meant to give you a mechanism to stay with the program when you've had difficulty. You should treat your commitment to Transition like a lifeline. Your ability to make and keep a total commitment for a ten-day period of time can really change your relationship to food. If you adhere to it completely, it works exactly as promised. It's just as important, however, not to use one slip-up as a reason to undermine your success. Some people say the ten days are amazingly easy. Others find they rebel against the structure. Whatever the case for you, if you go off, go back to one all-vegetable day, and then pick up where you left off.

10. **Exercise is essential to The Bloomingdale's Eat Healthy Diet.** If you are not already engaged in a sustained aerobic activity at least four times a week, you must begin to cultivate the exercise habit. During Days 1 to 5 of

the Transition phase, you need to walk briskly for at least twenty minutes daily. Starting at Day 6 you should increase your walking time so that your walk lasts forty minutes by Day 10 (if not sooner). This exercise rule is as critical to the losing process as the food- and water-related rules. If you already engage in sustained aerobic activity, you can continue with it and forego the walk; however, any day during Transition that you don't do your normal exercise routine, be sure to walk.

11. **Plan your food. This is, perhaps, the most important rule of all.** Concentrate on what you will be eating. Even if you don't usually cook, read the recipes and experiment with at least one or two of the dishes. The directions are geared to encourage even novice cooks. Think about what foods to buy for eating at home or to bring to school or the office, so you'll have appealing snacks handy. Plan ahead when you go to restaurants so that you'll know what you're going to order even before you get there.

12. **Do not be lulled into a false sense of security by an initial quick weight loss.** You must follow the plan exactly if you want to achieve the long-term results.

The Importance of Days 1, 2, and 3

The first three days of the Transition diet are a cleansing phase, designed to begin to reduce the level of cholesterol and fatty acids in your blood. They also cleanse your palate so your ability to appreciate a variety of flavors is enhanced.

During these days you will be eating only vegetables. This has several advantages for you, not the least of which is quick initial weight loss.

First, vegetables are extremely low in calories, but high in water content, vitamins, minerals, and fiber. They're filling and satisfy the need to experience a wide range of flavors and textures. Unlike highly restricted juice fasts, your all-vegetable days will not leave you feeling tired, weak, or hungry (see page 66 for possible exceptions).

Second, vegetables are remarkably free of fat. Consequently, they will help lower the total fat content of your diet as recommended in the Dietary Goals for the United States for better health.

Third, many vegetables are high in potassium and low in sodium. This is especially important during periods of rapid weight loss when your body's reserves of potassium tend to be depleted.

Finally, these first three days will give you an opportunity to explore fully the potential of vegetables as a major component of a new, long-term relationship with food. The recipes marked "V" contain only vegetables and will surprise you with their diverse and tempting meal suggestions (see Chapter 8). Vegetables provide the ideal mainstay of a well-balanced diet. Many of us are so accustomed to meat as the focus of a meal that we often ignore the healthy, versatile vegetable. Use these three days to discover the range of possibilities inherent in this most perfect food group.

BREAKFAST

It's best to start off your all-vegetable days with something solid and satisfying. So you're about to be introduced to the pleasures of a potato for breakfast. That's right, a potato! Potatoes are an amazingly wonderful breakfast food. They're filling, rich tasting, and full of important vitamins and minerals, including vitamin C and potassium. And, perhaps best of all, they stay with you; they'll keep you feeling full for hours. In addition, a medium-size potato contains only ninety calories.

The only possible negative is that potatoes take a while to cook. So, for a quick start to the day, bake three or four potatoes ahead of time. Then, in the morning, you can simply slice one in half, place it in a hot oven (400° F) for fifteen minutes, and—*voila!*—breakfast is ready. Now, obviously, you can't use butter or sour cream. Try substituting two teaspoons of your alloted two tablespoons of plain, low-fat yogurt. Or try a teaspoon of dijon or other zippy mustard. If you wish, serve your potato with a sliced tomato or a small portion of Ratatouille (see recipe, page 160).

If you prefer to save your potato for lunch or dinner, try a vegetable soup (see page 144) for breakfast. Again, it's filling and easy to prepare. Or, have half a potato for breakfast and save the other half for another meal. If you're not a breakfast eater, it's okay to continue to skip it. Some people just aren't hungry when they wake up. If you don't feel energetic in the morning, however, I suggest you revise your old habits and begin to eat breakfast. If you prefer to continue without breakfast, add a mid- or late-morning snack of vegetables so that you're not overly hungry for lunch.

LUNCH

Lunch for the first three days will consist of a large salad, a big bowl of all-vegetable soup, a combination of the two, or any all-vegetable dish you wish. Use the recipes in Chapter 8 for inspiration and feel free to improvise. Learning to combine vegetables to complement each other in flavor and texture is fun. Salads and soups are easy to prepare, so there's no need to fuss. Just concentrate on using ingredients that are fresh and appealing. Check the ingredients list on commercial soups to ensure that they have no fat. If the package doesn't contain this information, don't buy the soup. Also look for commercial soups that have salt listed near the end of the ingredients. If salt is among the first three ingredients listed, it is too salty for the diet.

If you eat lunch in a restaurant, stick to salad or a plain steamed vegetable plate—most restaurant soups are higher in fat and salt than those recommended for the diet. Any all-vegetable salad is fine, as long as you order it without dressing. Request vinegar and a lemon wedge on the side. If the restaurant doesn't have an entrée salad on the menu, ask for a double-size salad. Be careful when ordering vegetable main dishes in restaurants. They are frequently served with sauce, grated cheese, or are sautéed in oil. Restaurants are usually very accommodating when you make special requests. The better the restaurant, the more cooperative they're likely to be. Ask for plain steamed vegetables, with no added oil or butter or salt.

DINNER

For most of us, dinner is more than a meal, it's a social occasion. Dinner is our time to be with family and friends, or just to indulge in a solitary "wind down" from the pressures of the day. You'll be delighted to see how easy it is to prepare delicious meals using only vegetables. Select an entrée from the main dish recipes, like Broiled Eggplant, Cabbage Sauté, or Baked Acorn Squash. Make sure that you choose recipes marked "V," which indicates that they are all-vegetable. Of course, if you haven't had your potato for breakfast or lunch, you can use it as the focus of your evening meal.

Serve your entrée with a complementary salad. It's important to provide contrast via color and texture. Garnish your plate with cherry tomatoes and watercress. Begin the meal with a small serving of soup. Be creative.

If you prefer to keep life simple, you can always repeat the recommended menu for lunch. Simply vary your soup and salad selections, so you don't get bored. But do check the recipes for easy suggestions. Variety is important to keep you feeling satisfied. Some recipes, like the one for acorn squash, simply require putting something in the oven.

It's best to avoid eating dinner out, especially during the first four days of the diet. If you do eat out, use the strategy recommended for lunch, and substitute your vegetable entrée for lunch that day. If you know ahead of time that you'll be going to a restaurant, you might want to save your baked potato for that meal. After Day 5 it's easy to eat out. But before then, especially at dinner, you might feel more satisfied if you can have a potato along with your steamed vegetables or salad. It's also wise to have a bowl of vegetable soup at home, before you leave. It's much easier to stick to your resolve if you're not hungry!

Experiment with the vegetable recipes. You'll enjoy discovering the variety of satisfying possibilities they suggest and you'll also see how easy it is to cook with no added oils. Preparation and cleanup are much easier for vegetables, too —another bonus.

SNACKS

If you haven't used them in a recipe, you may add half an apple and two tablespoons of plain, low-fat yogurt to any meal, or eat them separately as a snack from Day 1 through Day 8. In addition, you can eat raw and cooked vegetables from the "Unlimited" list (page 75) anytime you're hungry. Raw red peppers and carrots are particularly satisfying when you're craving something sweet. Soup makes a great bedtime snack. Remember, after Day 6 you can eat up to eight ounces of Priority Dairy products as a snack if you haven't eaten them at mealtime.

The Transition Phase— Prototype All-Vegetable Menus
DAYS 1, 2, AND 3

The following are suggested menus. You are free to make up your own, as long as whatever you eat is all-vegetable and you limit yourself to one potato a day. Remember to use only recipes that are marked "V" in Chapter 8 and to follow Rule 7 (page 50) for cooking techniques.

Note: ''R'' indicates that the actual recipe can be found in Chapter 8.

DAY 1

Breakfast:
   Potato with 2 teaspoons plain, low-fat yogurt
   Sliced tomato

Lunch:
   Gazpacho (R)
   String Bean and Carrot Salad (R)

Dinner:
   Baked Acorn Squash (R)
   Steamed Vegetables (R)
   Mixed green salad with Easy Mustard or Oriental
      Dressing (R)

Snack:
   Raw and cooked vegetables, as desired
   ½ apple and remaining plain, low-fat yogurt

> *Nutritional information*
> *for the entire menu:*
> *Calories: 820*
> *Protein: 38 grams (18% of calories)*
> *Carbohydrate: 158 grams (77% of calories)*
> *Fat: 4 grams (4% of calories)*

DAY 2

Breakfast:
   Ratatouille (R) with potato

Lunch:
  Zucchini Soup (R)
  Mixed raw vegetable salad (include lettuce, cucumber,
    carrots, red and green peppers, celery, sliced beets,
    and pimientos) with Creamy Vinaigrette (R)

Dinner:
  Broiled eggplant slices with Easy Tomato Sauce (R)
  Steamed asparagus with Easy Mustard Dressing (R)

Snack:
  Raw and cooked vegetables as desired
  ½ apple cut up and mixed with remaining plain, low-fat
    yogurt

> *Nutritional information*
> *for the entire menu:*
> *Calories: 902*
> *Protein: 44 grams (20% of*
> *calories)*
> *Carbohydrate: 177 grams*
> *(78% of calories)*
> *Fat: 2 grams (2% of*
> *calories)*

DAY 3

Breakfast:
  Potato with 2 teaspoons dijon or Pommery mustard
  Sliced tomato

Lunch:
  Carrot and Turnip Soup (R)
  Spinach Salad (R)

Dinner:
  Zucchini Soup (R)
  Cabbage Sauté (R)
  Broiled tomatoes

Snack:
  Raw or cooked vegetables as desired
  ¼ apple (¼ apple is in one serving of Cabbage Sauté)
    with remaining plain, low-fat yogurt

---

*Nutritional information
for the entire menu:
Calories: 905
Protein: 38 grams (17% of
calories)
Carbohydrate: 177 grams
(78% of calories)
Fat: 5 grams (5% of
calories)*

DAYS 4–10

Beginning with Day 4, you'll be adding the remaining food groups, one by one. It's important to note that each day is different in the number of servings from any given group. For example, you'll be eating two grains on Day 4, but only one grain on Day 5. Each day is fully described below, with a sample suggested menu. Or, you may follow the menu plan in "Ten Days at a Glance" by choosing selections for a stated food group from the "Permissible Exchanges" list on pages 75–79. You must adhere to the serving size and the number of servings permitted each day. The exchanges allow flexibility and individual preferences. Vary your choices to ensure a good nutritional balance. Some people like to follow the suggested menus exactly, others prefer to make substitutions from the "Permissible Exchanges" list. Just be sure to follow Rule 1, which tells you to eat exactly the number of servings per food group permitted each day, and you won't go wrong.

DAY 4
Add grains
Follow the meal plan for the first three days exactly,
but with two additions.

Breakfast:
The same as Days 1–3; potato with vegetables as
desired

Lunch:
Vegetables as desired (i.e., salad and soup)
Add one slice of whole-wheat or whole-grain bread,
such as rye or pumpernickel, or select one item from
the "Grains" section of the "Permissible Exchanges"
list. You may use approximately one tablespoon of 1
percent-fat cottage cheese as a spread for your bread.

Dinner:
Soup and salad as desired
Add ½ cup cooked rice, preferably brown. Mix with 2
teaspoons of your plain, low-fat yogurt allotment to
give it a creamy taste. If you prefer, you can
substitute 1 scant cup cooked pasta for the rice. Serve
it with Vegetable-Based Spaghetti Sauce (R), but
forego the cheese.

Snack:
Raw and cooked vegetables as desired
½ apple cut up and mixed with remaining plain, low-fat
yogurt

*Nutritional information
for the entire menu:
Calories: 993
Protein: 40 grams (16% of
calories)*

Carbohydrate: 197 grams
(79% of calories)
Fat: 5 grams (4% of
calories)

DAY 5
Add poultry or fish

Breakfast:
   The same as Days 1–4

Lunch:
   A whole-wheat pita pocket stuffed with shredded
   cabbage, lettuce, peppers, chopped vegetables, and
   tomato slices. Flavor with lemon juice and mustard.
   Have small portions of soup and salad *if* you still feel
   hungry.

Dinner:
   Broiled 3-ounce chicken breast without skin, steamed
   vegetables, and salad. Try marinating the chicken
   breast in fresh lemon and lime juice to give it a
   delicious flavor. Be sure to choose vegetables of
   different colors and textures.
   Note: Eat only one grain selection today so that you
   don't increase your calorie count too quickly.

Snack:
   Raw and cooked vegetables as desired
   ½ apple cut up and mixed with remaining plain, low-fat
   yogurt

Nutritional information
for the entire menu:
Calories: 1096
Protein: 83 grams (30% of
calories)

*Carbohydrate: 173 grams
(63% of calories)
Fat: 8 grams (6% of
calories)*

DAY 6
Add dairy

From Day 6 on, you must have 8 ounces of Priority
Dairy products (see page 77) every day. Priority
Dairy products are the only dairy products permitted
during Transition except for the small amounts of
low-fat (1 percent) cottage cheese indicated on some
menus and in some suggested recipes. In addition,
Priority Dairy products will constitute your primary
source of dairy consumption at all times on the
program because these three items (skim milk,
low-fat buttermilk, and plain, low-fat yogurt) have a
significantly higher calcium content than other low-fat
dairy sources, including low-fat cottage cheese. If you
want to continue having a potato for breakfast, or if
you skip breakfast, be certain to add a Priority Dairy
selection to another meal or have it as a snack.

Breakfast:
¾ cup hot or cold whole-grain cereal (such as oatmeal,
Wheatena, Grape Nuts, Shredded Wheat, or Puffed
Rice) with 4 ounces skim milk

Lunch:
Half a toasted whole-wheat bagel or whole-wheat
English muffin, spread with 1 tablespoon 1
percent-fat cottage cheese
4 ounces plain, low-fat yogurt mixed with chopped raw
vegetables and flavored with chives

Dinner:
  Broiled 4-ounce fish fillet (choose sole, fluke, haddock,
    or similar). You can marinate the fish in lemon or
    use a splash of teriyaki sauce. Serve with salad and
    Basic Vegetable Sauté (R).

Snack:
  Raw and cooked vegetables as desired
  ½ apple cut up and any remaining Priority Dairy
    products if not eaten as suggested in the above
    menu.

> *Nutritional information*
> *for the entire menu:*
> *Calories: 1005*
> *Protein: 68 grams (27% of*
> *calories)*
> *Carbohydrate: 154 grams*
> *(61% of calories)*
> *Fat: 13 grams (12% of*
> *calories)*

DAY 7
Add citrus fruit
  Eat your citrus fruit at breakfast or during the day. Do
    not save it for after dinner.

Breakfast:
  Citrus fruit (orange, ½ grapefruit, or tangerine)
  ¾ cup hot or cold cereal (see Day 6) with 4 ounces
    skim milk

Lunch:
  Soup
  Chef salad with 3 ounces white meat turkey (no other
    meat or cheese)

Dinner:
   1 cup cooked pasta with Zesty Tomato Sauce (R)
   Green salad

Snack:
   Raw and cooked vegetables, as desired
   ½ apple with 4 ounces plain, low-fat yogurt

---

*Nutritional information
for the entire menu:
Calories: 1024
Protein: 63 grams (25% of
calories)
Carbohydrate: 175 grams
(68% of calories)
Fat: 8 grams (7% of
calories)*

DAY 8

Breakfast:
   Same as Day 7

Lunch:
   A whole-wheat pita pocket stuffed with shredded and
      chopped vegetables as per Day 5
   Serve with salad and/or soup if you feel hungry

Dinner:
   Tuna-Stuffed Potato (R)
   Salad
   Steamed Vegetables (R)

Snack:
   Raw and cooked vegetables as desired
   ½ apple and any remaining Priority Dairy products

> *Nutritional information*
> *for the entire menu:*
> *Calories: 1020*
> *Protein: 71 grams (28% of*
> *calories)*
> *Carbohydrate: 166 grams*
> *(65% of calories)*
> *Fat: 8 grams (7% of*
> *calories)*

DAY 9
Add dessert

Breakfast:
  Same as Day 7

Lunch:
  Ratatouille (R) with potato
  Salad

Dinner:
  Scallop Kabobs (R)
  ½ cup cooked brown rice
  Salad

Dessert:
  Select any fruit from the "Permitted: Once-a-Day" list
    (page 78)

Snack:
  Eliminate the half an apple on Day 9 and Day 10. For
  'snacking, reserve your breakfast or dessert fruit, or
  snack on raw or cooked vegetables. In addition, you
  can snack on up to 8 ounces of Priority Dairy
  Products if you haven't used your full allotment
  during the day.

---

*Nutritional information
for the entire menu:*
Calories: 1100
Protein: 91 grams (33% of
calories)
Carbohydrate: 175 grams
(64% of calories)
Fat: 4 grams (3% of
calories)

DAY 10

Breakfast:
 Same as Day 7

Lunch:
 ½ small cantaloupe with 3½ ounces plain, low-fat
  yogurt
 1 slice whole-wheat or whole-grain toast
 Salad, if desired

Dinner:
 Chicken and Mushroom Risotto (R)
 Salad

Dessert:
 Broiled Banana. Peel, then slice a banana in half
  lengthwise. Sprinkle with fresh lemon and lime juice
  and cinnamon. Place under broiler for 7–10 minutes.
  Serve with a dollop (½ ounce) of plain, low-fat
  yogurt. If you prefer, you can select one portion of
  any fruit you desire (see pages 78–79).

Snack:
 Same as Day 9

*Nutritional information
for the entire menu:
Calories: 1057
Protein: 65 grams (24% of
calories)
Carbohydrate: 179 grams
(68% of calories)
Fat: 9 grams (8% of
calories)*

Potential Problems and Pitfalls

For most people, Transition represents a significant and abrupt change in eating habits. It's not surprising, then, that there are a variety of reactions you might experience. Most of them will be positive. A few may be uncomfortable. I want to discuss all the possible problem spots, even those that are rare, so you'll be well prepared. As you read this section, keep in mind that most people really have very little trouble.

The most common problems occur within the first three days. If you don't already have a high proportion of fresh vegetables in your diet, you're likely to feel bloated and a bit gassy during the all-vegetable days. Don't worry, you're not gaining weight from vegetables! The bloat will disappear by about Day 5, and the gassy feeling along with it.

Occasionally people are troubled by diarrhea. If that happens to you, eat cooked, rather than raw, vegetables. Feel free to take an over-the-counter medication to settle your stomach. It's rare to need it, however. If the condition persists, cut back on the vegetables you're eating and add plain rice. Potato and rice will get you over your difficulty and you can pick up the program with the next day in sequence as soon as your stomach quiets down. Sometimes people are troubled by constipation. Take a natural fiber laxative until your system adjusts. It may take you a few days, but adjust you will. If either condition persists, consult your doctor.

Another consequence of eating vegetables (and drinking six to eight eight-ounce glasses of water a day) is that you're going to feel the need to urinate more frequently. Women tend to be troubled by this more than men. But it's very common, and it's likely to last well into the ten days. It, too, will subside as you adjust. Be sure to keep drinking your water. It's worth it!

I've already warned you about the complications that are caused by caffeine (see Rule 4, page 48). If you feel tired or headachy or irritable, it may be linked to a withdrawal from, or a continued use of, caffeine. Even people who don't have a coffee habit frequently experience feeling light-headed, or a bit shaky, at one point or another during the first three days. It's important to know that these feelings are normal and generally pass quite quickly. If you should feel tired, carrots and red peppers are both good pick-me-ups because they're naturally sweet. *If you feel weak, you're probably not eating enough. Don't "binge diet." Eat!*

If you know that you are eating the full allotment of food on the program, and you have persistent feelings of weakness or tiredness, you may need to add a bit of protein before Day 5. Don't struggle with yourself or think that you're failing in any way. Trust your body to tell you what you need. If the feelings are pronounced, just eat some water-packed tuna or a few ounces of chicken without any skin. You won't need much, and it will make you feel better.

One common pitfall is to become "scale crazy." It's fine to weigh yourself every day if you understand that your weight will fluctuate at times for no apparent reason. It would be very motivating to monitor a rapid weight loss by watching the needle on your scale descend day after day. Unfortunately, that's not how it usually works. Weight loss happens in spurts. You will drop three pounds at a time, even five, or seven. But then you'll step on the scale one morning and see a two-pound gain. The most common reaction is to panic; to assume the diet isn't working. Relax. That's how the diet works. You are witnessing the weight-loss process—which includes a range of fluctuations. Obviously, if you haven't been faithful to the program, you need to pay more attention to the evidence on the scale. But if you are adhering to the diet, ignore the scale. I tell Workshop participants to believe their clothes, not their scales. Scales can be inaccurate or reflect conditions that aren't significant. Clothes never lie. If your pants are tight after they've been roomy, something may be amiss. Otherwise, don't let a momentary variation on a scale rock your confidence. Here's a good place to warn you that some people truly are what I call "slow losers." Most often, slow weight loss is caused by not following the rules exactly, particularly the exercise rule. There are those, however, who will not see the quick initial weight loss promised. If you are one of them, stick with it. You may lose more slowly, but you will lose steadily.

Any other problems you have are likely to be connected to the five things I mentioned in Chapter 1: commitment, food, water, exercise, and support. You need to have all five in place for you to get the most out of Transition. Together they work to keep you feeling great while you're losing weight rapidly. Drop one, forget just one of them, and you're more likely to have a problem.

The one final area that may cause concern is emotional. The truth is that Transition is more difficult to think about than to do. The most common reaction is to feel high. However, depending on your own individual circumstances, there are a wide range of emotions that may surface. You need to be willing to feel whatever you feel at this time, and not act on it. You may feel angry, resentful, or sad.

For example, Howard, a sixty-five-year-old executive who had retired just before he went on Transition realized that what he was feeling was grief. "It's like I'm in mourning for all the food I'm not eating," he told his group in their second session. "I feel like I've been giving up a lot of things recently: my work, my office, the luxury of having a personal secretary. And now my regular six o'clock cocktail, too." Howard's mood lifted the next morning. He not only successfully lost the thirty pounds he had targeted, but also never went back to his sundown cocktail—even after he got on Personalization!

Don't anticipate problems. You're unlikely to have any, and if you do, they're unlikely to be really troublesome. After all, you're not on a diet now and I'll bet that you're occasionally tired, weak, headachy, irritable, even bloated or gassy. The question is, How often are you high, energetic, excited, optimistic, bouyant, and eating delicious food—guilt free? Because once you weather any problems that do pop up, that's how you're going to feel!

The Transition Phase—
Ten Days at a Glance

DAYS 1, 2, and 3

Breakfast:
　Potato with vegetables, if desired

Lunch and Dinner:
　All vegetable selections; choose recipes marked "V"

Snack:
　Vegetables as desired
　½ apple and 2 tablespoons plain, low-fat yogurt if not
　　used in recipes

DAY 4
Add grains

Breakfast:
  Potato with vegetables, if desired

Lunch:
  Vegetable selections
  1 item from the "Grain Exchange" section of the
    "Permissible Exchanges" list (see pages 76–77)

Dinner:
  Vegetable selections
  Grain exchange

Snack:
  Vegetables as desired
  ½ apple and 2 tablespoons plain, low-fat yogurt if not
    used in recipes

DAY 5
Add poultry and fish

Breakfast:
  Potato with vegetables, if desired

Lunch:
  Vegetable selections
  Grain exchange

Dinner:
  Vegetable selections
  Poultry exchange or fish exchange

Snack:
  Vegetables as desired
  ½ apple and 2 tablespoons plain, low-fat yogurt if not
    used in recipes

DAY 6
Add dairy

Breakfast:
  Grain exchange
  Priority Dairy exchange (see page 77)

Lunch:
  Vegetable selections
  Grain exchange
  Dairy exchange

Dinner:
  Vegetable selections
  Poultry exchange or fish exchange

Snack:
  Vegetables as desired
  ½ apple and unused Priority Dairy exchange (if any)

DAY 7
Add citrus fruit

Breakfast:
  Grain exchange
  One piece citrus fruit
  Priority Dairy exchange

Lunch:
  Vegetable selections
  Poultry exchange or fish exchange

Dinner:
  Vegetable selections
  Grain exchange
  Priority Dairy exchange (if not used as a snack)

Snack:
  Vegetable as desired
  ½ apple and unused Priority Dairy exchange (if any)

DAY 8

Breakfast:
  Same as Day 7

Lunch:
  Vegetable selections
  Grain exchange

Dinner:
  Vegetable selection
  Poultry exchange or fish exchange

Snack:
  Vegetables as desired
  ½ apple and unused Priority Dairy exchange

DAY 9
Dessert fruit

Breakfast:
  Same as Day 7

Lunch:
  Vegetable selections only

Dinner:
  Vegetable selections
  Poultry exchange or fish exchange
  Grain exchange

Dessert:
Choice of once-a-day permitted fruit

Snack:
Vegetables as desired
Unused Priority Dairy exchange (if any)

DAY 10

Breakfast:
Same as Day 7

Lunch:
Vegetable selection
Fruit exchange
Priority Dairy exchange
Grain exchange

Dinner:
Vegetable selection
Poultry exchange or fish exchange
Grain exchange

Dessert:
Choice of any fruit

Snack:
Vegetables as desired
Unused Priority Dairy exchange (if any)

	DAY									
	1	2	3	4	5	6	7	8	9	10

Number of Servings per Day
(✓ means item is permitted)

	1	2	3	4	5	6	7	8	9	10
Vegetables (unlimited) raw and cooked as desired from the "Unlimited" list	✓	✓	✓	✓	✓	✓	✓	✓	✓	✓
potato (once-a-day)	✓	✓	✓	✓	✓	✓	✓	✓	✓	✓
Grains (see Appendix) bread crackers miscellaneous grains	0	0	0	2	1	2	2	2	2	3
Animal Protein (3–4-ounce serving) poultry or fish	0	0	0	0	1	1	1	1	1	1
Priority Dairy (total 8 ounces) skim milk—4 ounces low-fat buttermilk—4 ounces plain, low-fat yogurt—4 ounces	0	0	0	0	0	2	2	2	2	2
Fruits (1 piece)	0	0	0	0	0	0	1	1	2	3
citrus							✓	✓	✓	✓
permitted once-a-day									✓	✓
limited (3 servings per week)										✓
Snack (if not used at meals) ½ apple	✓	✓	✓	✓	✓	✓	✓	✓		
2 tablespoons plain, low-fat yogurt	✓	✓	✓	✓	✓	✓	Any unused Priority Dairy			
vegetables as desired	✓	✓	✓	✓	✓	✓	✓	✓	✓	✓

VEGETABLE LISTS

Unlimited
artichokes
asparagus
bean sprouts
beets
broccoli
brussels sprouts
cabbage
carrots
cauliflower
celery
cucumber
eggplant
green beans
greens (beet, chard, chicory,
    collard, kale, spinach, etc.)
leeks
lettuce (all varieties)
mushrooms
okra
onion
parsley
peppers
potato (one per day)
radish
squash (all varieties: acorn,
    butternut, spaghetti, one
    medium squash per day)
tomato
turnip
zucchini

Limited
(After Transition Phase is completed: no more than ½ cup
    serving, once a day)
beans and peas
(dried or cooked, kidney,
    lima, navy, soy, split, etc.)
corn
sweet potato
tofu
yams

Note: Peas, beans, and tofu may be used as a protein exchange.

How to use the chart: When a prototype menu calls for 3 ounces of tuna, for example, you may substitute 3 ounces of any other fish, poultry, or meat (after Transition) from the animal protein group. Likewise, if cereal is called for, you may make a "grain exchange" and use 1 slice of bread or 1 cup cooked pasta instead. An entry from one group is not exchangeable for an entry from another group (for example, tuna is not exchangeable for oatmeal). The exchanges apply only *within* the various groups. Permissible Exchanges are not necessarily equivalent in nutritional and caloric value. They have been developed to facilitate menu planning and to provide satisfactory portions. Consequently, it is important to vary your choices to ensure a well-balanced diet.

Note: You may use beans, peas, and tofu (listed under Limited Vegetables) as an animal protein exchange after Transition—or during Transition if you are a vegetarian.

Grains
Cereals (¾ cup serving)

Cream of Wheat	oatmeal
farina	Puffed rice, wheat (1 cup)
Grape Nuts (½ cup)	Shredded Wheat
Nutri-grain (varieties without sugar)	Wheatena

*Breads (1 slice is a single serving)**

bagels (½ bagel is a single serving)	whole wheat (½ whole-wheat English muffin)
pumpernickel	whole grain
rye	whole-wheat pita pocket (1 medium-sized pita pocket is a single serving)

*Note: Men can usually continue to lose weight quickly utilizing 2 slices as a single serving—but not during Transition.

Crackers
Finn Crisps (4 crackers)
Norwegian Flat Bread
(1 slice)
rice cakes, unsalted
(2 crackers)
Wasa Crisp Bread (2 slices)

whole-wheat breadsticks
(2 sticks)
whole-wheat matzos
(1 cracker)

Miscellaneous Grains
½ cup cooked brown rice
⅔ cup cooked bulgar wheat

½ cup cooked millet
1 cup cooked pasta

Animal Protein
Fish (3–4-ounce serving)

bass	mackerel	snapper
bluefish	mussels	sole
clams	oysters	swordfish
crab	salmon (water-packed	tuna (water-packed or
flounder	or fresh)	fresh)
fluke	scallops	trout
haddock	scrod	turbot
lobster	shrimp	

Poultry (3–4-ounce serving, without skin)
chicken   turkey

*Meat (3–4-ounce serving—lean, all fat removed, after Transition no
more than once a week, one of the following)*
beef   lamb   veal

Dairy
Priority Dairy (After Day 6 of Transition: 2 4-ounce servings per day)

Note: During Stabilization (see Rule 6, page 87), if you do
not choose to have your optional Miscellaneous Dairy
Selection, you may have up to 12 ounces of Priority Dairy.

low-fat (1 percent) buttermilk
plain, low-fat (1.5 percent) yogurt
skim milk

*Miscellaneous Dairy (After Transition is completed you may have one
extra, optional dairy serving per day in addition to two 4-ounce
servings per day of Priority Dairy.)*
cheddar cheese (1 tablespoon grated)
low-fat (1 percent) cottage cheese (3 ounces)
feta cheese (1 ounce)
hoop cheese (3 ounces)
Parmesan cheese (1 tablespoon grated)
romano cheese (1 tablespoon grated)

Note: Cheddar is a high-fat cheese that should be used sparingly
to add flavor to recipes. You can use other hard cheeses (i.e.,
Swiss, Muenster, Monterey Jack, etc.) in the same way. If a
cheese isn't listed, the permitted quantity is 1 tablespoon
grated for hard cheeses, or 1 ounce maximum for soft
cheeses.

Fruit
(After Day 10 of Transition: a maximum of 3 servings per day
from the following lists. Do not have the same fruit twice in
one day.)

Permitted (once a day)
apple
berries (1 cup)
cantaloupe (½) or 5″ wedge of honeydew, crenshaw,
watermelon, etc.
fresh fruit salad (1 cup)
grapefruit (½)
mango (⅔ cup)
nectarine
orange
papaya (½)
peach
pear
pineapple (1 cup, unsweetened)
plum (2 small or 1 large)
tangerine

Limited (total of 3 servings per week)
apricot (2 small)
banana
cherries (1 cup)
figs (2 small)
grapes (1 cup)

NOT PERMITTED

---

all oils and fats (vegetable and animal), including butter,
  margarine, shortening, lard, etc.
all prepared salad dressings, except those without oil
prepared sandwich spreads such as mayonnaise, Miracle Whip,
  etc.
sugar in any form (fructose, dextrose, sucrose)
syrups, including molasses and honey
jams and jellies
egg yolks (egg whites are permitted)
avocados, olives
all nuts and extracts of nuts, including peanut butter
all seeds (pumpkin, sunflower, etc., except very small amounts,
  such as the sesame seeds on a breadstick)
cream, whole milk, sour cream, flavored yogurts, plain yogurt
  with more than 1.5% fat, cottage cheese with more than 1%
  fat, cheese (except as indicated on the "Permissible
  Exchanges" list)
canned or frozen fruit with added sugar
juices, including fruit and vegetable (except as indicated in
  recipes)
non-dairy substitutes
all meat and meat substitutes not found on the "Permissible
  Exchanges" list, including pork, ham, sausage, bacon, salami,
  etc.
prepared dessert toppings such as Cool-Whip
cake, cookies, and other baked goods, fresh or frozen
candy, soda (including dietetic)
gum, including dietetic (breath mints are permitted, in very
  limited quantities—not more than two a day)
fried foods of any sort, including potato chips, corn chips, etc.

snack crackers and corn—caramel corn, cheese corn, etc. (except those crackers on the "Permissible Exchanges" list)

Note: Air-popped popcorn, without butter, is permitted as a snack after the Transition phase is completed. Limit: 2 cups a day, 3 times a week.

5

The Stabilization Phase

By now you undoubtedly feel that incredible sense of joy that accompanies a loose waistband. You've probably taken off at least five, if not twelve or more, pounds. You know that the promises I made about the benefits of Transition are true: You're feeling great and loving food, really delighted in your appreciation of subtle taste sensations.

One of Bloomingdale's top personnel executives told me a story that illustrates that moment of recognition when people really see the benefit of Appetite Training for themselves. It happened just before she went on Stabilization, on Day 9 of Transition. She was having a snack with her niece. The niece was eating ice cream while Mandy was savoring a fruit salad, her first in over a week.

Mandy said that there was this huge, "decadent" strawberry that she'd saved for her last bite. When she tasted it, it was so indescribably sweet and delicious that she wanted her niece to taste it. Her niece thought the berry was "okay" but couldn't understand why Mandy was swooning. "I suddenly realized," Mandy said excitedly, "that that's what you'd been talking about. I wasn't even interested in Becky's ice cream. I was so bowled over by my strawberry that it was all I cared about. I'd been dreaming about fruit, not ice cream. And, wonder of wonders, the fruit I tasted surpassed my fantasy. I hadn't even noticed the craving for ice cream had gone. It was the first time I'd stopped and thought about how dramatically my taste sensations and desires had altered in only ten days." Isn't it great to be able to identify with that experience?

Remember Dennis, the meat-and-gravy-lover I mentioned earlier? He took a little longer to realize how profoundly his preferences had been affected. He marveled that he was never hungry during Transition, and that, yes, he did enjoy what he was eating—but he'd clung to the idea that he'd prefer his old favorites. Well, a few weeks into the Stabilization phase, he called to relate that "it" had finally happened. He'd gone to a dinner at a friend's who'd served his old favorite: roast beef with lots of gravy. "I was sitting there thinking, this tastes so rich, so really heavy. And I caught myself in the thought. It hit me that this was me sounding like you; me thinking roast beef was 'heavy.' I realized I'd just as soon be eating fish. In fact, I thought about a broiled snapper I'd had the night before, fresh and not overdone. I had to laugh at myself: the convert!"

Wherever you are in your own progress with Appetite Training, as along as you have completed Transition, you are ready to enter the next phase, Stabilization. It's not as revolutionary as Transition, but it's no less important and no less effective.

The Process of Stabilization

Remember Rule 12 of Transition? It warns you not to be lulled into a false sense of security because of a rapid weight loss. To maintain your loss, and continue to lose, you need to make your new habits second nature. The way to do that is to follow the rules for Stabilization.

Stabilization is a much more flexible phase. It's designed to provide you with an ideal balance of both structure and flexibility. It's the bridge between the revelations of Transition and the reality of Personalization.

Depending on how much weight you need to lose, you might be on Stabilization for one month, or one year, or more. I consider one month the minimum period for this phase, even if you reached your goal in Transition, because you need to live on the program for at least that time to have it "stabilize" for you; to make it your way of life. In fact, for Appetite Training to be fully successful, Stabilization must become the blueprint for your basic eating habits. Personalization is simply a method for individualizing Stabilization. For the most part, you will have the latitude you need to live happily, within the guidelines for Stabilization.

That latitude includes cheating. I want to talk about this right up front because you and I both know that unless you're one of a rare minority, you're going to cheat. There will even be times when you should cheat. You can't live a full life and never cheat. It's unrealistic to expect it of yourself, and unnecessary to attempt it. The less you do it, the faster you'll lose—and the easier it will be, by the way. But if you put yourself under too much pressure, you're much more likely to fall prey to the all-or-nothing syndrome that is the source of most diet failure. Guideline 9 (page 91) covers cheating. It calls for an all-vegetable day, just as on Transition. It's an easy mechanism to get you back in touch with your trained appetite immediately. Just as it's part of the process to cheat, so it must become automatic to adhere to Guideline 9. Don't get into a pattern of cheating one day and eating vegetables the next. The advice at the end of this chapter will help you know when to give in and when to resist. For now, just know that permanent weight loss means that you have to be able to accommodate the real you living in the real world. The wonderful thing about Stabilization is that it encompasses so much great eating that cheating will not be a major issue.

By the way, let me pass on a hint that I use in my Workshops. After Transition, it's often helpful to include just one grain or protein serving in an all-vegetable day. You don't have to, but if it makes it easier for you, I think it's advisable. The point of an all-vegetable day is to use it as a tool to return you to the program. If a minor adjustment makes it easier to use, it's well worth it.

Before you read the guidelines, take a moment to visualize your Ideal Body Image. Relax and get your image clearly in front of you. After you read this paragraph you should close your eyes and concentrate on it. You need to recognize that you are now significantly closer to making that image a reality than you were just ten short days ago. You've traveled much further than the time span would indicate. Entering Stabilization means you've completed the Transition phase. You're not only many pounds closer to your goal, but also that much more equipped to achieve it. You know now that your natural appetite loves the food that will make your ideal you real.

This may sound a bit strange, but when you close your eyes and conjure up your Ideal Body Image, be certain to have the image say "thank you" to you. You deserve it.

Guidelines for Stabilization

The guidelines for the Stabilization phase are simple, especially since you've been living with them already in Days 9 and 10 of Transition. Stabilization is the program you should follow until you reach your goal weight and have stayed there at least one month. It's very important to continue to drink at least six eight-ounce glasses of water daily and to exercise four to six days a week. Most people continue to lose quickly and steadily on the following program:

1. **Eat vegetables every day, preferably both raw and cooked.** Choose at least three different vegetables, the greater the variety the better. Include a dark green leafy vegetable daily. Vary the color of the vegetables you eat to ensure a good balance of vitamins and minerals. Remember that if you cook them, do so briefly to retain their maximum nutritional value. You can eat one potato a day, but from now on you should treat it like a grain. Therefore, never eat a potato in a meal with grains, bread, or cereal. (See rules for potatoes on page 94.)

2. **Eat two to three servings of whole grains daily.** Cereal in the morning is one good source. Brown rice, pasta, or whole-grain bread should be part of lunch and/or dinner. Be careful about portions. Three-quarters of a cup of cereal, half a cup of cooked rice, or one cup of cooked pasta are the appropriate quantities. For men, two slices of bread equal a single serving; for women, it's only one. Men need to use their judgment about serving sizes more than women. Men should try to balance their desire for fast weight loss against their need to feel satisfied. If one slice of bread satisfies, it's obviously preferable to two. If half a cup of rice leaves you hungry, it's okay to have a bit more. Just remem-

ber, there's no fooling the scale. Unfortunately, women have less leeway. In general, women can gain weight more easily than men because they require fewer calories. They therefore need to be more strict with serving sizes. Remember, grains should be eaten at mealtime. Do not "save" grains for after-dinner snacking.

3. **Don't worry about getting "enough" protein.** Because the vegetables, grains, and dairy products you'll be eating contain substantial amounts of protein, you can keep legumes, chicken, or fish (or lean meat once a week) selections to a minimum. I recommend that you eat one serving of legumes, chicken, or fish each day, although it isn't necessary to have one serving every day as long as you maintain a high vegetable intake. For chicken or fish, a serving is three to four ounces; for legumes, half a cup, cooked, is a serving. Chapter 8 contains a number of hints on how to add legumes to recipes, so be sure to read it thoroughly. The serving size is crucial, as is the cooking method (see Rule 7, page 50). Avoid all fatty meats, not just for your waistline, but for your health as well. Get in the habit of using meat as a part of a recipe (as in the Chicken and Mushroom Risotto recipe, page 176). Read Oriental cookbooks for inspiration. Just be sure to substitute wine and/or broth for the oil used in stir frying until you reach your goal (see Guideline 4, page 120). It is also helpful to cultivate a taste for legumes as a healthful protein source. Beans and peas have almost no fat, are very high in fiber, and consequently are an excellent alternative to fish and meat protein. After Transition, you can add them to soups, vegetable sautés, and casseroles to make easy, one-dish suppers (see Chapter 8 for suggestions).

4. **Avoid all added oil, butter, margarine, cream, sour cream, mayonnaise, and fats of any kind.** Remember, fats are the single greatest source of hidden calo-

ries—120 per tablespoon! You needn't worry about having enough, because fish, chicken, most dairy products, and certain grains and vegetables contain some fat. Wouldn't you rather have a piece of bread with a bit of cottage cheese (1 percent fat, of course)? After ten days of the Transition phase it will be easy for you to cook delicious meals without these unnecessary calories. And if you use no fats in your cooking, it helps to compensate for the added fat you're bound to get when you eat out. No matter how carefully you order, there will undoubtedly be hidden fat in restaurant food. Don't worry about it; just be careful at home and be as specific as you can when you order in restaurants.

5. **Eat a maximum of three pieces of fruit a day.** One should be citrus, not just because it's high in vitamin C, but also because citrus fruits are dependably low in calories. If you still have a lot of weight to lose, keep your fruit selections to two. If you should have a sweet attack, eat three fruits, rather than something with sugar. Pineapple is the best cure for a sweet craving I've found. Be sure to let your fruit ripen before you eat it. It contains a few more calories, but it will be much more satisfying. Buy it before you plan to eat it, and let it stay outside the refrigerator for a few days. Apples are an exception. Refrigerate them immediately. Avoid all dried fruit, until you reach your goal. Then, use it sparingly, as a condiment to enhance another dish (i.e., a few raisins in the cavity of a baked apple). I don't think it's worth the calories myself, but if dried fruit enhances a dish for you, go ahead.

6. **Have eight ounces of low-fat dairy products a day from the Priority Dairy foods on the "Permissible Exchanges" list.** Skim milk (not 1 percent fat milk!), low-fat buttermilk (great for making soups creamy), and plain, low-fat (1.5 percent) yogurt are especially important for women. This is because women tend to

lose calcium during and after menopause, and this can lead to osteoporosis. Consequently, it's important to build up calcium intake when you are young to counteract this tendency as you age.

In fact, I agree with the many medical authorities and nutritionists who recommend that women include a calcium supplement in their diet. Five hundred to 1,000 milligrams of calcium daily is what is usually recommended. Calcium in the form of calcium carbonate is recommended because this preparation offers the highest percentage (40 percent) of elemental calcium. However, it's best to consult your physician before starting a calcium supplement. It is possible to develop kidney stones if too much calcium is consumed.

In addition to the eight ounces of Priority Dairy foods, you may choose one additional, optional dairy exchange per day that does not have priority status (or you may choose an additional priority exchange). This will enable you to plan a wide variety of appealing menus.

Be very aware of the fat content in the dairy foods you eat. Look for the fat content on the label. Only 1 percent fat is permitted for cottage cheese, 1.5 percent for yogurt. Don't be fooled by part skim milk cheese. The other part is high-fat and that means high calories. Avoid using cheese when you are having a protein selection. Occasionally using grated cheese on vegetable selections will satisfy a craving for cheese flavor.

Note: Don't eat cheese and then sit down to a meal. When you eat it, include it in your meal. We've been conditioned to think cheese is a healthy snack. In fact, it's a high-fat, high-calorie trap. One little cracker with cheese tends to lead to another. Carrots are for snacking. Cheese should be used in small amounts (see "Permissible Exchanges") to enhance the flavor of a meal. Always avoid high-fat cheeses like brie. Instead, choose a low-fat chevre (goat cheese), feta cheese, or a bit of grated Parmesan or cheddar for flavor.

7. **Get a feel for the right balance in your food selection.** This is the key to enhancing your weight loss while on Stabilization. Rather than create hard-and-fast rules for you, I've indicated flexible guidelines that allow you to create a variety of appealing alternatives for yourself. The purpose of the Stabilization phase is to teach you to eat, not to diet. The more you choose to eat vegetables as the focus of your meals, the faster the weight will come off. As an alternative, get into the habit of using grains as the focus, with fish or chicken as a side dish (i.e., half a cup of brown rice with chicken, fish, or legumes, or a bit of chicken, seafood, or legumes in a pasta sauce or risotto), because the combination does make a very satisfying meal. Pasta with vegetable-based sauces is an ideal dinner choice if you've had a protein selection at lunch. If you can forego the Parmesan cheese, so much the better; you're saving thirty calories per tablespoon.

It's perfectly okay to go for a day or two with no fish or chicken selection, because you're getting protein in grains, dairy, and vegetables. If you've eaten in a restaurant, and have had a larger than recommended serving of fish or chicken, for example, avoid them the next day. Don't go overboard, however. Eating well-balanced meals will increase your sense of well-being and satisfaction. One small serving of protein, eight ounces of Priority Dairy Products, three servings of grains, three fruits, and lots of vegetables make an ideal pattern (for examples, see the "Prototype Stabilization Menu," pages 92–93, and the "Sample Stabilization Menus," pages 94–107). Varying the pattern occasionally is also good for avoiding the boredom that can occur when you fall into a set routine.

8. **When eating in restaurants, be sure to ask how particular selections are prepared.** It's fine to ask whether the spinach has been sautéed in olive oil, or if the primavera sauce on the pasta has butter or cream in it (you can bet it does, unless it's a tomato-based sauce). Request that fish be broiled dry, that vegetables and salads be served plain, with lemon and/or vinegar on the side. You can always order the exact amount of what you want (i.e., three ounces of turkey in a chef salad or sandwich) because restaurants are very aware of portion sizes. So don't be shy, be specific! Here are some specific hints for smart ordering.

   Japanese restaurants offer a wide range of good choices. Sushi, for the initiated, is an excellent option. Kappa maki, which is simply cucumber rolled in rice and seaweed, is delicious. Order it with a few pieces of raw fish sushi. Request lemon wedges to squeeze into your soy sauce. It dilutes the soy sauce, thereby cutting down on the sodium. Seafood sukiyaki and yosenabe are also fine on Stabilization. Both are fish stews (yosenabe also contains chicken) that contain lots of vegetables and cellophane noodles, both of which are low in calories. Chicken and fish teriyaki may also be ordered. Request that they go light on the teriyaki because it does contain both sugar and sodium.

   Italian restaurants also offer lots of good choices. Beware of vegetable selections, since olive oil is used lavishly. Instead, order clams possilipo, or mussels marinara. If you feel hungry, ask to have them served with half an order of pasta. Either would be better than traditional white clam sauce, which is made with lots of olive oil. Red clam sauce, on the other hand, is tomato-based, and an acceptable choice. Spaghetti with marinara sauce is fine, as are *zuppa de pesce* (an Italian fish stew) and any broiled or poached fish. Broiled chicken or veal chops are also usually prepared acceptably. The portion will undoubtedly be too large, however. Take half home, or indulge yourself, and avoid chicken or fish the next day.

In American and French restaurants, simple broiled fish and chicken, large salads, vegetables that are steamed without added oil or butter, pastas with tomato-based sauces, and other plain dishes of this sort are the best selections. Chinese restaurants tend to use more oil than is desirable. Most offer steamed fish, which is delicious, and they are happy to steam vegetables as well, instead of stir-frying them. When you order a stir-fried dish, request that they use less oil. Be explicit when you ask. Some selections are cooked to order. Ask which are. Indian, Thai, and Mexican food all offer interesting possibilities since they have so many vegetable and bean choices. The problem again is oil. If you order something that looks very oily, don't be shy about using a teaspoon to skim off the oil you can see.

The best advice I can give you is to plan ahead. Whenever possible, choose restaurants where you know you can get cooperation ordering. If unsure, call ahead and discuss the possibilities with the maître d'hôtel before you even get there. Restaurants today are used to such requests and are in the business of serving you, the patron. When you find yourself somewhere where there are slim pickings, order a salad and baked potato. If that's not possible, and the temptation is too great . . .

9. **If you cheat, enjoy it, but don't use it as an excuse to undermine your success.** Chances are, you will "fall off the wagon" occasionally. That's not setting you up for failure, it's just telling you what to expect. You will cheat. Know it now. It probably won't even taste that great to you. If you do cheat, get back on the track with an all-vegetable day. If you find yourself craving sweets again, be sure to cut them out completely, in-

cluding fruit, for at least two or three days. The strategy is to provide flavor interest in an area outside the one giving you trouble. So, when in doubt, or in trouble, eat vegetables. If you find yourself getting into the habit of cheating, go back to the Transition phase and take yourself through the whole ten-day program. Most Workshop participants, especially those with large weight-loss goals, have found that it's helpful to do that periodically. You will need less reinforcement the longer you are faithful to the Stabilization phase.

One last word about cheating—be sure to notice how you feel right after the meal, and the next morning. Listen to your body; it's a sensitive machine that will talk back when given the wrong fuel.

10. **Finally, eat.** If you're used to it, eat three meals a day. Snack frequently—whenever you're hungry (on vegetables, obviously). At the risk of repeating myself, plan your food—especially before eating out. It helps in a restaurant to know what you are going to order. Look for recipes that you can adapt. If you feel deprived, buy a papaya or a mango.

Prototype Stabilization Menu

Breakfast:
  1 potato, or
  1 cereal, or
  1 bread (spread with 1 tablespoon low-fat cottage cheese)
  4 ounces Priority Dairy exchange
  Fruit (once-a-day list, emphasize citrus)

Lunch:
  Soup and/or salad
  1 fish, poultry, legume, or dairy selection, and/or
  1 bread, cracker, or grain selection
  Vegetable selections

Dinner:
  Soup and/or salad
  1 fish, poultry, or legume (if you haven't had it at
    lunch) and/or
  1 grain, bread, or cracker selection
  Vegetable selections

Dessert:
  Fruit

Snack:
  Raw or cooked vegetables as desired
  1 fruit
  Up to 8 ounces of Priority Dairy choices if you haven't
    already used them during the day.

This is your potential daily food selection before you reach
your weight-loss goal. To maximize your continuing weight
loss, it's best not to eat one of every option. For example, it
is not necessary to have a protein serving every day, nor
should you have a protein serving at a meal with a dairy
selection. Although you are permitted a protein, dairy, and
up to three grain selections, it is best to avoid having the full
allotment. Instead, follow a pattern that conforms to the
following guidelines, until you have reached your goal:

QUICK WEIGHT-LOSS GUIDELINES

2 grain selections
2 Priority Dairy selections
1 additional dairy selection
1 fish, poultry, or legume selection (3–4 ounces), optional
3 or more servings of varied, unlimited vegetables (keep your
  vegetable intake very high on days you do not have an animal
  protein selection)
2 fruits

The beauty of the Stabilization phase is that it is very flexible and can be adapted to your day-to-day needs, but it can be confusing at first. You are permitted the full selection pattern indicated in the Prototype Menu above. You may trim it back to the more limited pattern recommended in the Quick Weight-Loss Guidelines. It's helpful to think of the full Prototype as the maximum you should eat and the Quick Weight Loss Guidelines as the minimum.

Listen to your body. Now that you've had the experience of feeling great while eating only vegetables, you know that a bowl of soup and a salad will keep you satisfied. Surely, all-vegetable meals will help speed your continuing weight loss. Still, for optimum nutrition, you need to incorporate a variety of foods and give your body a continuous source of high-quality fuel. So, use your judgment, and let your natural appetite response (not your emotions or your habits!) be your guide.

The rules for potatoes are:

1. Treat your potato as a grain exchange
2. One potato per day
3. Never eat potato with bread, cereal, or grain

Use the following Sample Stabilization Menus to help you get a sense of the desired pattern needed to ensure healthy continuing weight loss.

Sample Stabilization Menus

You will see when you read the nutritional listings following each daily menu that the number of grams of protein, carbohydrate, and fat vary from day to day. For example, the menu for Day 1 contains only 51 grams of protein, slightly less than the RDA for the average man of 56 grams, while the menu for Day 8 contains 73 grams of protein, well over the RDA. What's most important, however, is the average daily intake.

These menus will help give you an idea of how to follow Guideline 7 of Stabilization—the one that is concerned with a proper dietary balance. Keeping your diet well-balanced is essential to healthy weight-loss. Use the nutritional listings in these sample menus as your guidelines to ensure that your body is well nourished over a period of time.

Note: "R" indicates that the actual recipe can be found in Chapter 8. Snacks to ensure sufficient Priority Dairy are indicated. Vegetable snacks should be eaten as desired. Men may increase portion sizes for grain selections as indicated in Guideline 2 (page 85).

DAY 1

Breakfast:
   ¾ cup Shredded Wheat
   4 ounces skim milk
   ½ grapefruit

Lunch:
   Ratatouille (R)
   Baked potato
   Green salad

Snack:
   4 ounces plain, low-fat yogurt with cinnamon

Dinner:
   Basic Vegetable Soup (R)
   Spaghetti with Zesty Tomato Sauce (R)
   Cucumber Salad (R)

Dessert:
   Broiled Banana (page 65)

*Nutritional information
for the entire menu:
Calories: 1194
Protein: 51 grams (17% of
calories)
Carbohydrate: 234 grams
(78% of calories)
Fat: 6 grams (5% of
calories)*

DAY 2

Breakfast:
    ¾ cup cooked oatmeal
    4 ounces skim milk
    1 orange

Lunch:
    Carrot and Turnip Soup (R)
    Spinach Salad (R) with
    1 tablespoon grated Parmesan cheese

Dinner:
    Italian Clam Soup (R) with slice garlic toast
    Large mixed salad
    Steamed asparagus

Dessert:
    1 cup blueberries with
    4 ounces plain, low-fat yogurt

*Nutritional information
for the entire menu:
Calories: 1178
Protein: 65 grams (22% of
calories)*

*Carbohydrate: 198 grams
(67% of calories)
Fat: 14 grams (11% of
calories)*

DAY 3

Breakfast:
 ¾ cup Shredded Wheat
 4 ounces skim milk
 Slice melon

Lunch:
 Hearty Cabbage Soup (R)
 Chef salad with 3 ounces turkey
 1 slice whole-wheat toast

Snack:
 4 ounces plain, low-fat yogurt

Dinner:
 Spaghetti and Broccoli (R)
 Green salad

Dessert:
 1 cup strawberries

*Nutritional information
for the entire menu:
Calories: 1105
Protein: 66 grams (24% of
calories)
Carbohydrate: 181 grams
(66% of calories)
Fat: 13 grams (11% of
calories)*

DAY 4

Breakfast:
  1 slice whole-wheat toast spread with 1 tablespoon
    low-fat cottage cheese
  4 ounces skim milk
  ½ banana

Lunch:
  Carrot and Turnip Soup (R)
  ½ Baked Acorn Squash (R)
  Broiled tomato
  ½ cup cooked brown rice

Dinner:
  Broiled flounder
  Ratatouille (R)
  Endive salad

Dessert:
  Fruit salad of ½ cup raspberries and ½ banana, sliced,
    mixed with
  4 ounces plain, low-fat yogurt

*Nutritional information
for the entire menu:
Calories: 1178
Protein: 63 grams (21% of
calories)
Carbohydrate: 191 grams
(65% of calories)
Fat: 18 grams (14% of
calories)*

DAY 5

Breakfast:
  ¾ cup cooked oatmeal

4 ounces skim milk
½ grapefruit

Lunch:
Cold Zucchini Soup (R)
Basic Vegetable Sauté (R) mixed with
½ cup cooked brown rice and
1 ounce feta cheese

Snack:
4 ounces plain, low-fat yogurt

Dinner:
Sole with Tomatoes (R)
Baked potato
Large green salad
Steamed carrots

Dessert:
Slice watermelon

Nutritional information
for the entire menu:
Calories: 1148
Protein: 58 grams (20% of
calories)
Carbohydrate: 202 grams
(70% of calories)
Fat: 12 grams (9% of
calories)

DAY 6

Breakfast:
1 cup puffed rice
4 ounces skim milk
1 cup strawberries

Lunch:
  Basic Vegetable Soup (R)
  3 ounces cottage cheese with apple slices
  ½ whole wheat bagel

Dinner:
  Mixed salad with tomato
  1 cup cooked pasta with asparagus and Zippy Mustard
    Dressing (R)

Dessert:
  1 cup fresh pineapple chunks with
  4 ounces plain, low-fat yogurt

---

*Nutritional information
for the entire menu:
Calories: 1138
Protein: 67 grams (24% of
calories)
Carbohydrate: 186 grams
(65% of calories)
Fat: 14 grams (11% of
calories)*

DAY 7

Breakfast:
  1 slice whole-wheat toast spread with 1 tablespoon
    low-fat cottage cheese
  4 ounces skim milk
  1 orange

Lunch:
  Cool Cucumber Buttermilk Soup (R)
  Baked Acorn Squash (R)
  Sliced tomato salad

Dinner:
  Chicken and Mushroom Risotto (R)
  Steamed broccoli
  Carrot Salad (R)

Dessert:
  1 cup strawberries

> *Nutritional information
> for the entire menu:
> Calories: 1000
> Protein: 54 grams (22% of
> calories)
> Carbohydrate: 178 grams
> (71% of calories)
> Fat: 8 grams (7% of
> calories)*

DAY 8

Breakfast:
  ¾ cup cooked Wheatena
  4 ounces skim milk
  ½ grapefruit

Lunch:
  Tuna-Stuffed Potato (R)
  Raw carrot and red pepper slices

Snack:
  4 ounces plain, low-fat yogurt with ½ apple

Dinner:
  Spaghetti and Broccoli (R), with
  1 tablespoon grated Parmesan
  Tomato and onion salad

Dessert:
1 cup pineapple chunks

---

*Nutritional information
for the entire menu:
Calories: 1161
Protein: 73 grams (25% of
calories)
Carbohydrate: 188 grams
(65% of calories)
Fat: 13 grams (10% of
calories)*

DAY 9

Breakfast:
½ bagel-spread with 1 tablespoon low-fat cottage cheese
4 ounces skim milk
1 slice honeydew melon

Lunch:
Eggplant and Rice Casserole (R)
Green salad

Dinner:
Cool Cucumber Buttermilk Soup (R)
4 ounces broiled scrod
Steamed green beans
Sliced tomato salad

Dessert:
Sliced mango

---

*Nutritional information
for the entire menu:
Calories: 1036
Protein: 64 grams (25% of
calories)*

*Carbohydrate: 159 grams
(61% of calories)
Fat: 16 grams (14% of
calories)*

DAY 10

Breakfast:
  1 cup puffed wheat
  4 ounces skim milk
  ½ grapefruit

Lunch:
  Zucchini Soup (R)
  Pita stuffed with shredded raw vegetables and 3 ounces
    water-packed tuna moistened with two teaspoons
    plain, low-fat yogurt and lemon juice

Snack:
  4 ounces plain, low-fat yogurt

Dinner:
  Stuffed Onions (R)
  String Bean and Carrot Salad (R)
  ½ cup cooked brown rice

Dessert:
  ½ papaya

*Nutritional information
for the entire menu:
Calories: 1005
Protein: 64 grams (25% of
calories)
Carbohydrate: 158 grams
(63% of calories)
Fat: 13 grams (12% of
calories)*

DAY 11

Breakfast:
  ¾ cup cooked Cream of Wheat
  4 ounces skim milk
  1 tangerine

Lunch:
  Hearty Cabbage Soup (R)
  Baked potato
  Baked Butternut Squash (R, see Baked Acorn Squash)
  Green salad

Snack:
  4 ounces plain, low-fat yogurt with cinnamon

Dinner:
  Broiled chicken marinated in mustard and lemon
  Broiled tomatoes
  Steamed broccoli

Dessert:
  1 pear

*Nutritional information
for the entire menu:
Calories: 1181
Protein: 64 grams (22% of
calories)
Carbohydrate: 202 grams
(68% of calories)
Fat: 13 grams (10% of
calories)*

DAY 12

Breakfast:
  1 slice pumpernickel toast spread with 1 tablespoon
    low-fat cottage cheese

4 ounces skim milk
½ cantaloupe

Lunch:
  Hot Zucchini soup (R)
  Broiled Eggplant (R)
  Stewed tomatoes
  Mixed lettuce salad

Snack:
  4 ounces plain, low-fat yogurt

Dinner:
  Herb-Broiled Scallops (R)
  Steamed escarole
  ½ cup cooked brown rice with 2 tablespoons plain,
    low-fat yogurt

Dessert:
  2 small figs

---

*Nutritional information
for the entire menu:
Calories: 1154
Protein: 72 grams (25% of
calories)
Carbohydrate: 185 grams
(64% of calories)
Fat: 14 grams (11% of
calories)*

DAY 13

Breakfast:
  1 slice rye toast spread with 1 tablespoon low-fat
    cottage cheese
  4 ounces skim milk
  1 slice crenshaw melon

Lunch:
  Carrot and Turnip Soup (R)
  Pita stuffed with shredded raw vegetables and ½ cup
    kidney beans moistened with two teaspoons low-fat
    yogurt and lemon juice
  String Bean and Carrot Salad (R)

Snack:
  4 ounces plain, low-fat yogurt

Dinner:
  1 cup cooked Spaghetti with Greek Tomato Sauce (R)
  Escarole and romaine salad

Dessert:
  1 peach

---

*Nutritional information
for the entire menu:
Calories: 1138
Protein: 54 grams (19% of
calories)
Carbohydrate: 217 grams
(67% of calories)
Fat: 6 grams (5% of
calories)*

DAY 14

Breakfast:
  ¾ cup Nutri-Grain cereal
  4 ounces skim milk
  1 orange

Lunch:
  Baked Eggplant (R)
  Broiled tomato
  Green pepper and carrot slices
  2 whole-wheat breadsticks

Snack:
4 ounces plain, low-fat yogurt

Dinner:
Basic Green Soup (R)
Scallop Kabobs (R)
Steamed vegetables

Dessert:
Baked apple

---

*Nutritional information
for the entire menu:
Calories: 1004
Protein: 60 grams (24% of
calories)
Carbohydrate: 173 grams
(70% of calories)
Fat: 8 grams (7% of
calories)*

If I Am Not Hungry, Why Am I Eating?

I've promised that you will learn to distinguish physical cravings from reflexive, habitual ones; that you will know when you should indulge a craving, and when you need to resist it. The method for learning how to do this is part of the process of Stabilization.

Breaking bad food habits is only the first step to ending diet failure. You know that much of the time, hunger has nothing to do with why you eat. It's after Transition, when your physical cravings are under control and you feel you have the whole problem solved, that you're going to start to experience a whole series of new cravings.

These new cravings aren't like physical ones. These new ones will feel like a compulsion to "cheat" even though you know that you're not hungry. It's a familiar sensation, I promise you. But it usually doesn't trouble people until Stabilization is pretty well under way. Before then, you're so intent on being good that your energy is well focused. As the diet becomes a natural part of your life, however, the other reasons you eat have room to surface.

I'm sure this isn't exactly news to you. You know your own food patterns by now. The distinction you may not have made before is to separate your physical cravings from your reflexive ones—in order to diffuse them. There's a simple procedure to help you do this.

First, there's the Craving Exercise, which helps expose the "anatomy" of the particular craving. Next, there's the strategy for Alternative Action, which works to diffuse the craving. Finally, there is advice for when, and how, to give into a craving.

You will have to examine your habits and emotions regarding food very closely. Through observing them, you open the way to change them. This doesn't happen instantly, but over time. And you'll always need reinforcement. In fact, when you reach Personalization, the skills you will have developed to deal with cravings become the rules for that phase.

The Craving Exercise is the first step. This is one of the most powerful tools of Appetite Training. I've learned that it takes Workshop participants a while to get used to using it, so I'll pass along a suggestion from one woman that might help you cultivate the habit. She copied the exercise on a three-by-five-inch card and carried it in her wallet. She said that even after she'd memorized the questions, the act of taking out the card and looking at it helped her "contemplate the craving, not indulge it." That's the secret. Once you learn to examine your cravings instead of act on them, you will have gained control over reflexive cravings! Whatever it takes to encourage you to use the Craving Exercise, do it. The sooner you use it, the sooner you'll reach your goal.

CRAVING EXERCISE

When you are hit by a craving for an unhealthy food, ask yourself the following questions:

1. What am I craving?
2. Am I actually hungry?
3. Did something happen to trigger this craving?
4. Would something else satisfy me? (Am I craving a sweet, something crunchy, etc?)
5. What is more important to me: my Ideal Body Image, or this momentary craving?

It's important to take yourself all the way through the exercise. Be sure to ask and answer each question. Frequently, just recognizing that you're not hungry, and that the reason you're craving ice cream is because you're disappointed, will be enough to diffuse the desire. At other times, you might discover that you do have a yen for something sweet, and fruit would satisfy. Using the craving exercise will help you examine your desires *before* you are tempted to act on them. You will discover, however, that there are times when you'll go all the way through the questions and the final answer will be that you care more about ice cream than your Ideal Body Image. What you need to do then is take an Alternative Action.

ALTERNATIVE ACTION

Part of the reason you eat is because it gives you something to do. It's active. It alleviates boredom. It makes you feel better to do something for yourself when you're blue. It gives you an outlet when you're angry. Trying not to eat when there's a desire to do so requires a strategy that recognizes this need to initiate action.

Before you give into a craving you should seek an alternative. *Delaying* an indulgence and doing something else is an essential strategy for altering reflexive eating. An active delay is much more effective than a passive one. Trying to wait it out often ends up focusing more attention on the food you're not eating. When you engage in a purposeful action, however, you most often divert your attention, thereby letting the craving pass.

What kind of action? For some, the telephone is the first line of defense. For one thing, it's offensive to hear someone chewing on the other end of the line. For another, just telling someone that you're blue, or angry, or feel like eating, helps. Other Alternative Actions might be walking around the block, cleaning out a drawer, writing a letter—or cooking! Cooking can be very effective because it's satisfying to be around food, even if you're not eating it.

Nancy, a young mother with three children under the age of ten, told me the following: "Before I took the Workshop, I hated cooking. It was a chore; something I couldn't escape. But then something clicked for me. I think it was when I made Zucchini Soup the first time. I just loved it. I couldn't get over the fact that I could eat as much of it as I wanted. I thought of it as 'my' food. Then I started to get excited. I made lots of different recipes, looking for ways to tempt myself. I was always cooking against the clock before. But once I saw that I could somehow designate it as a hobby, for myself, the time was there. What's really funny is that because I'd assumed the kids wouldn't like the food, they did. I started out serving them one thing, and my husband and me something else. It took two meals for them to demand equal treatment. If I had planned it as a strategy it probably wouldn't have worked! Anyway, now, when I have an urge to eat, I think, great, what should I cook?"

Don't be lazy about taking Alternative Actions. You'll need to motivate yourself the first few times. But then it will become a habit. Can you imagine how different your life will be when it's your reflex to take a walk when you feel nervous, instead of eating? If you think it can't happen to you, it's only because you're not willing to give it a try.

When to Give in to a Craving

There are times when you should indulge your desires. You need to be strict with yourself about when they will be, but it can undermine your long-term success if you have unrealistic expectations about what constitutes staying on the program. Eating foods that are off the diet is part of the process. Transition, Stabilization, and Personalization guidelines all offer advice about what's appropriate, and how to compensate when you do cheat.

It is appropriate to go off the program when you've gone all through your Craving Exercise, have taken an Alternative Action, have delayed the indulgence a fair amount of time, and you still want it, whatever it is. Don't spend a week thinking about chocolate cake. Eat a piece and get on with your life. Follow it with an all-vegetable day—and don't waste any energy on feeling guilty. Just be certain not to make it a pattern. Something sweet, every few days, will totally undermine your success and you'll find yourself addicted again in no time.

Stimulus/Response Eating

You won't be giving in to cravings often, and yet you will have them with some frequency. They won't be strong, or troublesome, just thoughts that you'd like to eat this, or that would taste good. What you need to do is become savvy about the nature of these passing thoughts and what causes them.

Reflexive cravings are caused by stimulus/response eating. It's useful to look at the stimuli that generate the response. Most often they are food as (1) a celebration/reward, (2) a sign of love, or (3) a leisure activity.

Food is your most frequent way of celebrating and rewarding yourself. When you want to celebrate a birthday, promotion, marriage, or just that it's Saturday night, you eat. If something goes wrong, you make up for it by rewarding yourself with food. But food is not simply a reward; it's one way you have to show people that you love them. (By the same token, not eating your mother's lasagna may be seen as a rejection of her!) It's also the best "time passer" known.

The objective isn't to never use food for the above purposes. What you need to do is to broaden your resources for celebrating and rewarding yourself, showing love, and spending time.

For example, Angela offered a great idea one night in a Workshop session for how she broke a long tradition in her marriage. "We're both great cooks," she told us, "and our ritual was that we'd each cook the other a feast of favorites for birthday celebrations. Well, it wasn't all that hard for me to create a sensational dinner of great food, on the program, for Jack's birthday. But I felt something was missing. I mean, I just felt I needed the equivalent of a chocolate soufflé. So Jack's dessert was a full-hour body massage. I heated the oil and everything. It was great. We both loved it! And let me tell you, am I ever looking forward to celebrating *my* next birthday!"

Interestingly, massage, facials, pedicures, and the like have all been mentioned frequently as desirable alternate rewards. There's a sensual, hedonistic aspect to them. Angela also said that she'd rediscovered the pleasures of a bath. "I noticed that when I got really low I'd crave rice pudding. Rice pudding was my mother's remedy for whatever was ailing us. I think it was the only thing she knew how to cook. There was something so infantile in that craving that it made me think about what the closest thing to the womb would be—and I came up with the bath. I take baths all the time now; when I'm depressed or disappointed, or even when I have time to kill. I love it. I play Chopin or Willie Nelson, depending on my mood. It's so relaxing. And there's no guilt!''

Food as a sign of love is more subtle. I wasn't kidding when I said that your mother might consider it a rejection of her if you turned down her lasagna. It's important to let those close to you know that if they really love you, they'll understand how important your commitment to this program is. Let them know that you know that they only want to please you, but that they aren't really doing what's in your best interest. This is harder for people who may look thin on the outside, but who think fat on the inside. To those who wish you well with cake and cream sauce, simply express your gratitude verbally, and eat what you choose to eat.

Finally, there's food as a leisure activity. It's not just that eating is fun and social. It's that it's so easy and available. Whenever you have a minute to kill, there's the temptation to spend that sixty seconds munching. Because we're hardly ever out of reach of food, this is an important habit to break. I keep a notebook with me so that I can write down odd thoughts or make notes to myself about work when I have extra time. Some people use knitting. Mystery readers are in luck because it's easy to take a paperback along with you. Still, there's nothing wrong with plain old relaxing. Try just letting yourself enjoy inactivity. It's okay to take a few minutes every once in a while to just stare into space. It can be very productive time. You never know what creative thoughts your mind might conjure up, given the chance!

These stimulus/response eating habits are so ingrained that they never disappear completely—nor should they. Still, you need to build your repertoire of responses to the everyday stimuli that lead you to eat. Remember, the power of a broken habit is that the process of breaking any pattern once makes it easier to do it on subsequent occasions. You need to be observant. Simply notice your behavior and recognize that you don't have to keep reacting the same way to the same situations forever.

Before we leave the subject of stimulus/response eating, I want to mention the everyday external stimuli that trigger reflexive cravings. I'm talking about the foods you see and smell as you go through the day. Walk down a city street on a summer afternoon and you'll see people eating ice cream cones. Pass by a bakery and the aroma of freshly made bread may tempt you. Turn on a television set or radio and you can't help being reminded of all the foods you're not eating. You must recognize that the desires aroused by these appetite teasers cannot be treated seriously. Your commitment is what will make the difference here. Once you behave as if your ideal body image is more important to you than a fleeting desire for ice cream, it will be easier to pass up the temptation the next time. Learn not to inhale when you walk by a bakery. Catch up on the newspaper during commercials. If you tell yourself that reflexive cravings don't deserve serious thought often enough, you'll eventually believe it—because you will have demonstrated that fact to be true. Ultimately, giving in to reflexive cravings doesn't make you happy. It makes you feel guilty, conflicted—and fat. Passing up the temptation will give you a deeper long-term pleasure. That's the truth.

You have the power to realize your most profound desires by making the simplest alterations in your customary *modus operandi*. It isn't hard to stare into space instead of munching a small bag of chips that might contain 500 calories. In two minutes you'd have forgotten that you'd even eaten them, but the results would sit on your hips for a long time. The alternative is a respite full of wonderful thoughts and fantasies.

6

The Personalization Phase

No matter how much I reassure people that "cheating" is part of the process, they're never really comfortable with that thought. For one thing, they worry about sliding back into old habits. For another, there's something undermining about thinking about maintaining a "diet mentality" that treats certain foods as cheats. In fact, if you can trust yourself around food, indulging when you choose to isn't cheating.

Alcohol is another area that makes new devotees to *The Bloomingdale's Eat Healthy Diet* pause and wonder. "It's amazing how little I've missed it," marveled Gregory, a forty-eight-year-old executive accustomed to two very dry "wind-down" martinis before dinner each night. "Still, I can't say I wouldn't love a drink or two," he added with a more than hopeful look in his eye.

The simple fact of life is that none of us (me included) wants to go through life totally excluding things that have given us pleasure in the past. Personalization, which is the third phase of Appetite Training, has been designed to en-

able you to include the treats most meaningful to you—both
as an everyday occurrence and as a sometime treat. Still, you
need to include them in a way that doesn't undermine the
effectiveness of your Appetite Training.

Getting Ready for Personalization

Personalization begins after you reach your goal. To ensure
that your new weight is stabilized, it's best to wait at least a
month before you begin to incorporate the Personalization
guidelines into your normal routine. Before that time, all
indulgences should be thought of as cheating on Stabilization. Consequently, they should be followed by an all-vegetable day.

You already know that when you were eating a diet of salt,
sugar, and fat, you craved foods containing them. And after
Transition and Stabilization, and a properly balanced diet of
body-enhancing foods, you craved "good" foods. So it may
seem at first that the question becomes: How much salt,
sugar, and fat can you consume without falling back into bad
habits? It's the wrong question.

Marjorie is a perfect example of the problems you might
have if you approach Personalization trying to fit in as many
of your old downfalls as you can. She lost forty-five pounds
in her Eat Healthy Workshop and was thrilled to be weighing what she had when she graduated from high school more
than twenty years earlier. She followed the program completely until she started Personalization and then a very interesting thing happened. She found herself indulging in just
those habits she'd broken, simply because she thought it was
now permitted. "I really discovered a lot about how tricky
my unconscious was," she told her group. "I wasn't even
craving anything and I'd watch myself compulsively eat food
I didn't really want. I realized that I didn't want to miss
anything I could have. If it was allowed, I felt cheated if I

didn't take advantage of it." Fortunately, Marjorie had been using the Craving Exercise and was very aware of her pattern. She caught herself as soon as the first few pounds showed up on the scale, had an all-vegetable day, and hasn't had a problem since.

The question you need to continue to ask yourself is: What am I really craving? Keep asking yourself that question, and your success with Personalization is virtually guaranteed. You'll be able to indulge, when you really want to, without risking a return to past addictions.

"You know," Ron, a twenty-seven-year-old buyer, told me recently, "when you used to talk about trusting yourself to know what you were really craving, I'd think, 'Oh sure, I'm the right one to trust!' I never imagined I'd be able to trust myself around food. I felt really scared before I started Personalization because I was so sure I'd blow it. But it was easy. Easy. I still can't believe this is me. I keep waiting for it to disappear. But anytime I've really indulged it's been no big deal. I'd be right on course the next day. I just naturally eat the way I eat now. It's incredible."

Let me explain further. I've set up guidelines for Personalization and, as the name implies, these guidelines are general and are supposed to be individualized. Each of us has different quirks of appetite. The phenomenon that amazes me is that in spite of the highly idiosyncratic nature of personal appetites, the pattern of cravings is fairly standard. That is, you will feel like having whatever it is (ice cream, alcohol, pastrami) fairly regularly. Every day there will be those stimuli that tend to trigger an eating response. For example, you might "want" ice cream when you pass someone eating an ice cream cone. Smell the aroma when you pass a croissant shop and it wouldn't be surprising to want a croissant. You'll discover, though, that the longer you go without these various "indulgences," the less you'll find yourself wanting them, even when those old triggers are pressed.

These predictable cravings are momentary reflexes.

They're the ones that have been ingrained in you through years of stimulus/response behavior. Go to the movies and you'll "want" popcorn. But once you pass the popcorn counter, and the picture starts, you'll forget about it. You can't treat these passing desires seriously. You already know that you're much happier, that you feel better, and that you certainly look better when you choose to crave your ideal body image more than your fleeting wish for a hot dog.

However, as I said before, there will be times when you really want that hot dog. You'll go all the way through your Craving Exercise, and the last answer will come up hot dog! Grown-ups in the real world have two-martini days. A vacation in France or Italy is undoubtedly more enjoyable if you don't make yourself order as carefully in restaurants as you do at home. There will be numerous times when the restrictions of Stabilization are unnecessary and too confining for the circumstances. How do you cope? How can you ease up without giving up?

The answer again is a question of balance. Basically, you'll be following the guidelines for Stabilization. To have a healthy, rewarding relationship with food you need to live your life on Stabilization (with some individual modifications I'll discuss in the Personalization guidelines). If you do, you will not experience strong cravings to do otherwise very often. That's the truth. So when you have a strong desire to do otherwise, enjoy it. Know that tonight you're going to have ice cream, and love it. Decide that this wine is worthy of more than one glass, and savor it. Don't agonize. Don't make deals with yourself. You needn't treat an indulgence like a cheat on Stabilization and have an all-vegetable day the next day. Reserve your indulgences for when you genuinely crave them, and you'll find yourself naturally in the proper balance.

It's hard to get used to the idea that you really will be able to trust yourself with food. You will. The longer you are on the program, the easier it will be. However, you need to be prepared for the persistence of stimulus/response reactions. Consequently, it's important to treat the Personalization guidelines like the rules for Transition. Follow them and I doubt you'll have much trouble.

Personalization Guidelines

1. **Always use the Craving Exercise when you're tempted by a craving.** Always ask yourself all five questions. Make certain that you conjure up a vivid picture of your Ideal Body Image when you get to Question 5. It can be tempting to think that you don't need to continue to monitor yourself in this way. But the process of breaking stimulus/response eating patterns is a lengthy one and you'll be more successful on Personalization if you're faithful to this rule.

2. **Always delay an indulgence.** This is one time when procrastination is good for you. If you're still dying for pizza after your Craving Exercise, take an Alternative Action. If that doesn't help, tell yourself you'll have it—tomorrow—*if* you still want it. Save your indulgence. Look forward to it. Save it up for a Saturday night. Look at it as a treat in the bank. The more often you delay it, the less often you'll want it.

3. **Never waste an indulgence out of laziness or expediency.** Don't eat anything off the program that you don't really want. If you're invited to a dinner party and aren't sure there'll be enough there for you to eat, have a bowl of vegetable soup before you leave home. It's easier to exercise restraint when you're not hungry.

Eat as little as possible in situations where the food is loaded with oil, mayonnaise, sugar, and the like. One ploy I use when I'm at intimate dinners and the hostess notices I'm not devouring her food with relish is to simply say that I've been feeling a bit queasy and think I'm better off eating very

lightly. No one wants a sick-to-her-stomach guest; the prod-
dings to just try the cream sauce cease.

4. **Be prepared for some adaptations that will affect
you daily.** Others will be once-in-a-while treats. You're
striving for an overall balance and it's not precise. If you
begin to tip too much toward Personalization, you'll start
having problems with increased cravings. Some common ad-
justments are as follows:

- Add one four-ounce glass of wine, one light beer, or two
  ounces of hard liquor up to five days a week. It's best not
  to get into the habit of having a drink every day, which
  is why I suggest limiting yourself to five days a week,
  maximum. Some studies indicate that modest amounts of
  alcohol (like those suggested) may actually reduce the
  risk of certain diseases. With an average of about 100
  calories or more for a drink, there's a trade-off involved.
  Remember, you could have a piece of bread, half a
  papaya with strawberries, or a potato for the same calorie
  count! Still, if you prefer the liquor, there's no reason
  not to have it. Obviously, there will be days when you'll
  want more than the amounts suggested above. You'll
  discover the latitude you have. But don't fall prey to the
  "Marjorie syndrome." Just because you can now have
  liquor as a matter of course, there's no need to drink
  more than you really want. Admit it, it hasn't been so
  bad feeling up and alert and energetic—even in the
  evenings!

- Add up to one tablespoon of oil or fat a day. Here again,
  you'll be getting 120 calories for each tablespoon, but
  there are times when it's worth it. For example, just one
  tablespoon of oil allows you to stir-fry the Chinese way
  much more successfully than with no oil. Two tablespoons of oil with some wine, broth, or sherry are sufficient for stir-frying enough for two to four people. If a
  recipe calls for more, cut it back and substitute more

wine or sherry. Some oils like sesame and walnut are very pungent and small amounts can add flavor to salad dressings. One teaspoon is all you'll need. I occasionally add a tablespoon or two of butter to a pasta sauce I'm making for company. You don't need one tablespoon per person, either. Just a dollop before you serve it makes certain sauces taste richer. I find this is particularly true with mushroom sauces. Now that you're used to food without oil and butter it would be criminal to cultivate the taste again. But as part of a recipe, a little may enhance a whole dish.

- The above principle holds for honey or sugar as well. Fresh fruit and plain, low-fat yogurt make a great dessert for trained appetites, but your kids and friends may appreciate something a bit sweeter. Just a teaspoon of honey (it's sweeter than sugar, but no less fattening for equivalent amounts) drizzled over broiled bananas, or mixed with the yogurt filling for a baked apple, will do the trick. Definitely do not get into the habit of sweetening things for yourself. Artificial sweeteners undermine Appetite Training even after you reach your goal. But a little sugar can sometimes go a long way. One place I use sugar is in cucumber salads. Just a pinch is all you need.

- Egg yolks may also be used from time to time as a facilitator in recipes. When a recipe calls for eggs, try substituting the whites, or perhaps one whole egg plus an egg white or two. Use your judgment. If a recipe serves four, and uses one egg yolk, it's no problem.

- You can loosen up a bit in restaurant ordering. If you eat out all the time you should be prudent on this one. Still, it is difficult to be in lovely restaurants and restrict yourself as judiciously as you have been. I would suggest you continue to avoid fried foods, cream sauces, and other overly rich items, except in the rarest of rare cases. But many chicken or veal dishes sautéed in wine, for example, have some oil or butter, yet are fine to order on Personalization. You don't need to eat all the sauce. If your order a dish with cheese, don't eat all the cheese. In general, choose wisely, since it's often difficult to leave something that tastes delicious. You needn't be so rigid that you limit your pleasure however. By the time you're on Personalization you'll discover that, just like Dennis, your natural appetite response will crave lighter fare. It's the old you who thinks you're wanting veal Parmesan, instead of veal marsala. As on Stabilization, if you have a large serving of protein in a restaurant, eat vegetables and grains the next day.

5. Continue to use the Prototype Stabilization Menu as your guidelines for planning meals, but you can begin to experiment with portion sizes. A whole bagel, instead of half. A more generous serving of rice or pasta. Grains three times a day, instead of the two you've been used to for quick weight loss. Don't increase too quickly, or you'll gain. But if you keep up with your exercise, you'll find that the longer you're at your goal weight, the more you can eat. It's infinitely better to increase your intake of desirable foods than to opt for the permitted extras. In other words, have the extra piece of bread rather than the drink. Choose an additional fruit over half of someone else's dessert. Remember that eating is good for you. Your body wants the nutrients available from wholesome food. You're cheating it if you feed it fat and sugar instead. You'll feel the difference.

6. Watch your pattern. Certain foods are addictive! A little sugar can lead to a lot. The idea that a little butter on your bread won't hurt is a lie: You can get used to the taste of butter on bread again in no time. It's a treat to have an indulgent meal with half a bottle of wine every once in a while. But what's every once in a while? If you find yourself craving problem foods, you're indulging too often. A glass of wine, a drink, a light beer, a slightly indulgent entrée, something stir-fried—these will be part of your life on an ongoing basis. It's the bacchanalia you've got to guard against. As a once-in-a-while thing, it's no problem. As a weekly event, you're headed for trouble. The best way to balance indulgences is to vary them. Make it something different each time. You might have a favorite dessert one night, and the next week, a slice of pizza. Then in a few weeks, a Chinese feast. In fact, most people find that once they get into the habit of delaying their indulgences, months can go by without going off the program to any great extent. You'll have so much invested in how you look and feel that it will seem a shame to lose momentum, or risk backsliding. The best part about *The Bloomingdale's Eat Healthy Diet* is that, unlike other diets, the longer you're on the program the less you'll want to go off it.

7. Remember, the Transition phase is always available to return you to your natural appetite response. After a vacation or a particularly celebratory time (Christmas season, a wedding in your family, etc.), you might find your weight up and your thoughts increasingly centered on food. Don't struggle with it. Go right back on Transition and you'll feel returned to yourself within the first few days. The longer you delay, the harder it will be. If you prefer, you can try an abbreviated version: As soon as you find yourself avoiding the scale, or notice your clothes are tight, have an all-vegetable day or two. Then use the Quick Weight-Loss Guidelines for Stabilization (page 93) until the extra weight comes off. If you have difficulty staying within those guidelines it's because you've become addicted again and you'll need to take yourself through the complete ten-day cycle. You'll need the whole process to clean out your system and give your taste buds a chance to become more sensitive. You might resist the thought, because the desire for sugar, salt, and fat is powerfully strong. Remind yourself of your experience this time. Recall your Ideal Body Image, or create a new one.

Appetite Training is like any life process; it requires

renewal. As a matter of fact, a good proportion of Workshop participants have reported that they go through Transition every two to three months as a matter of course. I go through the process about every three months. It makes me feel like I've been to a spa: cleansed and invigorated. I also find that it's a great antidote for depression. It gives you a project to tackle; an area in which you can take control and do something positive for yourself. Exercise, by the way, is another area of your life that works the same way. Exercise five days a week, and you'll love it. Slip back to three times a week and you'll find it harder to do. The fact is, your body has to depend on you to keep it in prime condition. And, at the risk of repeating myself, it's not just your body I'm talking about, it's your life!

Letting Yourself Succeed

You may have noticed that the human animal has a bewildering aversion to feeling great. We all explain this tendency differently to ourselves, but virtually everyone I've asked about this phenomenon is familiar with the pattern. Some people will explain it as the sensation of losing steam. "I'm a great beginner" is a phrase I've heard a lot in response to my queries.

This tendency isn't evident only in dieting. It permeates everything we do. You know how great you feel the first week in January when you're actually keeping your New Year's resolutions? If keeping them makes you feel so terrific, why fall back into your old bad habits? The most compelling explanation I've heard for the pattern is that it relates to the phenomenon of entropy.

Entropy is a measure of the amount of energy in a closed system. It explains the inescapable tendency of things to wind down as they approach a point of equilibrium. You may have noticed that as soon as things seem to come together in a project (or your life), they fall apart. That's entropy.

Yet, although that's the way things work when left to their own devices, it doesn't mean that human beings can't intervene. If you anticipate entropy, you can counteract it. You need to see yourself as an active force against entropy.

Understanding this role for yourself will provide you with an incredibly valuable tool as you live with Personalization. Once you've reached your goal, and begin to take a thin you for granted, there can be a reaction simply because you don't need to expend a lot of energy on the subject. You become less concerned with the whole matter. You'll tell yourself that you've got it under control and don't need to be so preoccupied. That's certainly true, but more than likely, what's going on has more to do with entropy than with success. It's when you're first really confident of your success that you need to be more vigilant. That's when the falling apart starts. Remember: Things come together, then they fall apart.

Learning that you can counteract entropy will have an impact on your life far beyond your success with *The Bloomingdale's Eat Healthy Diet*. Your relationships will have new dimensions if you grasp the power within you to revitalize them. Certainly your work will flourish when you take responsibility for infusing it with renewed commitment.

You don't have to succumb to a past pattern of losing steam. It's not hard to counteract entropy, especially since you've been in the mode of breaking past habits regarding stimulus/response eating. What's required is to continue those habit-breaking responses, even when you may not feel like it. *The Bloomingdale's Eat Healthy Diet* is actually an ideal opportunity to exercise all sorts of new habit-breaking responses. By being faithful to the program when you feel the desire to relax into past patterns, you set a new standard for yourself that has an impact on all your commitments.

Don't believe that things can't all go well. There's no rule of the universe that says nature always takes its course, or that every good event must be counterbalanced by a bad one. We all limit ourselves by our concept of reality and our desire not to tempt fate. You deserve to succeed. There's no reason why you shouldn't feel great and look your absolute best. You don't need the downers that come with excessive alcohol and a bad diet. You can enjoy food, life, and a permanently thin body—if you let yourself!

Dieting: The Problem You Used to Love to Worry About

Do you know that you used to love to worry about dieting? Even when you hated it, you loved it. Now that you're on Personalization, however, you might need to find some new problems to worry about.

I'm not kidding about this. I'm very serious. You used to worry about dieting to avoid other problems. I know. I watched myself cling to the problem for years. What I finally realized was that for some mysterious reason, I was keeping the extra weight on. I used to diet all the time anyway. There were years when I just didn't let myself be successful. As soon as the scale headed downward, I'd find myself eating. It took me quite a while to see and understand the way it worked. I think I can save you some time, in case it crops up again for you.

If you're already on Personalization, you may have forgotten what it was like, but it's useful to remind yourself of the syndrome. The pattern was to fill your time planning what you would and wouldn't eat. As you went about your day, doing all the things you had to do, there was a separate conversation that used to take place in your head. You know the conversation I'm talking about. It went something like:

If I have just this cereal for breakfast, I can have that Danish with some coffee at eleven o'clock. Or, maybe I'll skip the Danish and eat something really good for lunch, like pizza. I can always make up for it by going easy at dinner. But by the time dinner rolled around, the pizza was hours ago, and you'd be making deals with yourself about making up for it by eating just cereal for the next day's breakfast.

You probably still think about food frequently during the day. Notice, however, that the conversation in your head is probably a lot more positive these days. Useful planning and anticipating meals with pleasure is not the same as the "dieting: the-problem-you-love-to-worry-about" syndrome.

Worrying about food used to take you away from life and relationships. While you were sitting in a movie, instead of watching your favorite actor, bigger than life up there on the screen, you used to wonder whether or not to go get popcorn, and then make deals with yourself about what you'd have for dinner if you got it plain, rather than buttered. When your best friend poured out her heart about her problems with her twelve-year-old son, you'd be wondering how to convince her to go clear across town for lunch because you had a yen for Clancy's Irish Stew. While you walked around in your life, you had a series of events going on in your brain involving what you would and wouldn't, could and shouldn't eat.

If you're already on Personalization, that pattern is old news and will make you smile. But if you haven't yet started Transition (some people want to read the book all the way through before they make a commitment), it may be all too familiar. When you give that up, when you commit to being the thin person you want to be, you need other problems to fill the void. What happens on *The Bloomingdale's Eat Healthy Diet* is that some of that time is filled with the positive side of your new relationship with food. You still get to think about meals and plan your food and, yes, your indulgences. But being positive about your relationship with food takes nowhere near the energy that being negative used to absorb.

So be ready to take on some new challenges. You're going to have a new self-image and increased energy to go along with it. Your positive attitude about food will spill over into every other aspect of your life. When you give up dieting as the problem you love to worry about, you need to find some new problems. There's all that time to fill. So think about how to improve things at work or in your relationships. Concentrate on getting the political candidate of your choice elected, writing a best-selling novel, or whether or not your favorite team will make the playoffs. Look around you and find a useful problem to solve—because you won't have dieting to worry about any longer.

7

Answers to the Most Frequently Asked Questions About *The Bloomingdale's Eat Healthy Diet*

Q. What's the best way to speed my weight loss?
A. The answer is simple: Adhere to the program exactly. Most people make the mistake of thinking that eating less than what is recommended will speed their weight loss. In fact, if you cut back beyond the Quick Weight-Loss Guidelines for Stabilization, you may hinder your progress. Two things can happen. First, your body might react as if you were literally starving and slow its metabolism to conserve energy. Second, since you would not be eating a well-balanced diet, you might begin to experience troublesome cravings. You need to *eat* to lose weight. The only effective way to speed the process is to increase your exercise. You will not only

burn additional calories while you are exercising, but you may also continue to use energy at a higher rate for as long as twenty-four hours after each exercise session.

Q. If I feel tired should I eat more protein?
A. No. Protein is not your best energy source. Your body requires only small amounts of protein every day. If you feed yourself an excess of protein it will only get stored as fat. You need to examine when it is that you feel tired for clues to the source. If you find that you're tired during the day, chances are you're not eating well enough and often enough. It's common to feel an energy lag around 11:00 A.M. and 4:00 P.M. if you don't snack between meals. The best snacks, of course, are vegetables and Priority Dairy products. Another common source of a lack of energy is a lack of exercise. If you're eating enough, and exercising regularly, you should have energy to spare. If you don't, a check-up with your doctor may be in order.

Q. Don't I need some fat in my diet?
A. Absolutely. And, you're getting all the fat you need. Fish, chicken, grains, dairy products, and certain vegetables all contain fat. In addition, most of us don't prepare all our meals at home and consequently get more fat than we realize when we eat out, even if we're ordering very carefully.

Q. Why do you recommend exercising four to six days a week when so many experts say that three days a week is all you really need?
A. From my experience in Eat Healthy Workshops, I've seen that, generally, when people exercise three days a week, they need to push themselves to do it. However, when they add that extra day, they get addicted. The more often you exercise, the more often you will want to. In addition, every day you exercise is a day that you rev up your metabolism to burn extra energy.

Q. How soon can I add alcohol back into my diet?

A. My answer varies depending on the individual. You need to be scrupulously honest with yourself as you assess what's appropriate for you. In general, it's best to wait until Personalization and to follow the guidelines set forth in that chapter. However, if you're careful, you can begin to drink again before that, and for some people, knowing that they can drink occasionally helps them stay on the program. The qualifying factor should be how you yourself behave around alcohol. For some, the problem isn't the alcohol itself, but the behavior it triggers. For others, the idea of moderation around alcohol is just that, an idea. And then there are those who can have the occasional glass of wine, or Scotch and soda, without it leading to any undesirable effects. Where do you fall on the spectrum? And, how quickly do you want to lose weight?

For everyone, it is essential that there be no alcohol at all during Transition. I also advise that everyone, whether or not they need to lose weight, continue to abstain for as long as possible. The longer you're without it, the less you will miss it— and the easier it will be to establish a new relationship with it. If you're confident that you can drink in moderation (i.e., a glass of wine, a light beer, or one drink, no more than five days a week) and you haven't much weight to lose, you can begin to add alcohol about a month after you complete Transition. Watch yourself to see if the alcohol triggers any undesirable eating behavior. For those who have a more volatile relationship with it, I suggest waiting longer, and limiting it to two or three times a week for a significant period after you do resume drinking. If you still have considerable weight to lose, have alcohol only on special occasions, until you're on Personalization.

Q. How often can I eat sugar on Personalization?

A. There's no easy answer to this question. If sugar is a trigger food for you (a little makes you want a lot), the answer will be that you should eat it very rarely, or not at all. Beware especially of taking small bites of sweet things; you'll only perpetuate a sweet craving. However, if you have something sweet and don't find yourself craving more, you can probably enjoy an occasional dessert with no problem. The "how often" should be limited to how frequently you genuinely crave the flavor. Review the guidelines for Personalization to help you determine what's appropriate for you.

Q. How often can I go on Transition?
A. As often as you want as long as you don't use it to "binge diet." It's unlikely that you'll *feel* like going on Transition more than every few months. As I said earlier, I go through Transition every three months or so. For me, it's like going to a spa. I feel energized and refreshed by it. Many Workshop participants choose to repeat the Workshop after two or three months for the same reason. I recommend going through Transition at least once or twice a year as a way of breaking the small bad habits that inevitably crop up. If you want to speed your weight loss, or push yourself off a plateau, you can do it as often as every six to eight weeks without experiencing any problems.

Q. How often can I have an all-vegetable day?
A. You can have an all-vegetable day whenever you feel the need as long as you don't exceed one a week on a regular basis. You'll feel best when you eat a balanced diet. It's fine to have a few all-vegetable days to get you back on track if you've been having trouble. But if you develop habits that look like all-vegetables one day, and off the program the next, you'll know that you need the discipline of Transition and a commitment to Stabilization to break the pattern.

Q. Why do you show the number of people a soup recipe serves if the soup is "unlimited"?
A. It's just to give you an idea of how much it will make.

Any recipe marked "V" is unlimited. You can eat as much of it as you like. Just remember to be careful when you add beans, rice, or cheese to individual servings. Doing so changes its "unlimited" status.

Q. What are the biggest pitfalls during the Stabilization phase?

A. Overall, I'd say there are three:

1. Forgetting to eat a lot of vegetables. Some people are very careful about eating two or three grains and fruits, protein and dairy, but when you question them you find that they neglect to get enough vegetables. It's essential to continue to use vegetables as the mainstay of your diet. You need them for the fiber, vitamins, and minerals they offer, as well as to keep you feeling full and satisfied. If you aren't happy with the speed at which you're losing weight, ask yourself if you're eating enough vegetables. Remember, "less isn't better."

2. Forgetting your exercise and water. You need to continue to exercise four to six days a week, and to drink at least six eight-ounce glasses of water daily.

3. "Personalizing" Stabilization. Cheating on Stabilization is cheating. It needs to be followed by an all-vegetable day. As I said, you can have one grain or protein serving on your "all-vegetable" day once you're on Stabilization, but you need the discipline of that rule. If you adapt the program too early you'll lose the benefits of Appetite Training. The longer you follow the rules, to the letter, the easier the whole process will be.

Q. Is yoga a good form of exercise?

A. It's an excellent form of exercise but only as a supplement to an aerobic activity. Yoga is wonderful to ease stress and maintain flexibility. However, it does not get your pulse rate up and consequently does not work your heart muscle.

In addition to yoga, or any stretching exercises you do, you need to work aerobically at least four days a week.

Q. How is it possible not to feel deprived when you're not eating so many of the foods you love?
A. The most amazing part of Appetite Training is that *you won't crave what you don't eat.* You need to believe your experience on this one and not be undermined by your assumptions. If you make the leap of faith I discussed in the beginning of the book and just follow the rules of Transition, you'll discover that what I'm promising is true. If all you do is think about it, it won't work. Appetite Training can't work if you aren't willing to try it. The hardest part is thinking about it. Doing it is a breeze.

Q. How do I join a Workshop if I want more support than this book?
A. You can call the Eat Healthy office at (212)586-8038 or write to us at:

> Eat Healthy, Inc.
> 250 W. 57th Street
> New York, NY 10019

to find out if, or when, there will be a Workshop in your area or what other support material is available.

Q. What about taking vitamin supplements?
A. It is always recommended that people who go on any reducing regimen that might fall below 1,200 calories a day take a multi-vitamin/mineral supplement. It certainly can't hurt you. Unfortunately, many supplements contain unnecessarily high levels of certain vitamins and minerals—especially when you consider how rich *The Bloomingdale's Eat Healthy Diet* is nutritionally. My best advice is to look for a supplement with a very low dosage of Vitamin A: under 5,000 units is best (you'll be getting a diet that's very rich in beta caro-

tene on the program, which is the best way to get your Vitamin A). I also recommend that women take a *separate* calcium carbonate supplement so that they don't take it with nutrients that can inhibit absorption. Take your multi-vitamin in the morning after breakfast and your calcium at night. Unless you're in very skilled hands, "therapeutic" doses of vitamins and minerals are often wasted because they are in excess of your needs. The best way to get your vitamins is the way nature intended, in food. Follow the program and the way you look and feel will be proof of nature's sufficiency.

Q. My husband wants to make healthy changes in his eating habits, but he doesn't want to lose weight. How can he adapt the program?

A. The Transition phase is important for everyone who wants healthier eating habits, whether or not he or she needs to lose weight. It's important to break the food addictions that undermine good intentions. If your husband loses weight during those ten days, he can put it back on again easily by adapting Stabilization. The changes he should make involve increasing the quantity of complex carbohydrate (vegetables, fruits, and grains) and Priority Dairy. He should not increase the optional dairy or animal protein selections. In general, whole grains are the best foods to add for anyone who wants to gain or maintain his weight.

Q. What should I do if I am lactose intolerant?

A. Adult lactose (milk sugar) intolerance is extremely common. If eating dairy products results in abdominal bloating, flatulence, cramps, and watery diarrhea, you may be lactose intolerant. This means that your body is not manufacturing enough of the enzyme (lactase) needed to break down the lactose in your food.

Most people who are lactose intolerant can still tolerate small amounts of dairy products without any ill effects. Yogurt is a dairy product that is often tolerated. The portion sizes of the Priority Dairy Exchanges in *The Bloomingdale's Eat Healthy Diet* are small enough that they should not cause discomfort in anyone except those who are very lactose sensitive. There are also special products available for those who are lactose sensitive. Lacrose-reduced milk and cottage cheese are two of these products (but make sure they're skim and low-fat!). Lactase enzyme tablets as well as liquid lactase drops are also available in health-food stores and in pharmacies. The tablets are taken with meals or snacks and the drops are added to the milk twenty-four hours before it is consumed.

I hope the Bloomingdale's Eat Healthy Diet will give you as much pleasure, satisfaction, sense of accomplishment, and value as it has to the many people who have been through Eat Healthy Workshops.

Although I can't personally talk to each of you, I would like to support you as you go through the stages of the program and incorporate Effective Appetite Training into your daily life. We are constantly developing new recipes and hints at Eat Healthy and I believe they will help and support you.

_____

Dear Laura,

Name _____

Street Address _____

City _____ State _____ Zip _____

Telephone: Home_____ Work _____

Any comments about the diet you might care to make

_____

_____

_____

_____

_____

Please mail to:
EAT HEALTHY, INC. 250 West 57th Street, New York, N.Y. 10019 (212) 586-8038

8

Cooking Strategies
and Recipes

The pleasure of *The Bloomingdale's Eat Healthy Diet* comes from discovering how sensational a meal of wholesome food can taste. You can increase that pleasure substantially if you learn some simple techniques that allow you to cook your favorite foods without fattening additives such as oil, butter, cream, and sugar. In fact, many Eat Healthy Workshop participants report that they've taken a new interest in cooking because it enables them to indulge in the hedonistic delights of food, without paying the price of gaining weight.

Most of the recipes that follow are very simple. You don't need to spend your life in the kitchen to make delicious meals. Still, I've included a wide range of possibilities to tempt both novice and experienced cooks.

It's important to use the recipes as guidelines, and not rigid instructions. Vegetables vary in size, water content, and freshness. There are no hard-and-fast rules for how long they need to be cooked, or how much liquid they will give up. So you'll need to use your judgment and experiment a bit.

All the recipes contain specific advice and you'll soon find it becomes easy to judge for yourself.

Even if you think there's no way you could be lured into your kitchen unless it's to heat up something already prepared by someone else, read through this chapter. It's so easy to enjoy great food, guilt free, that you're really cheating yourself if you don't give cooking a try. Start with one or two soups and salad dressings to enjoy during Transition. Remember, all the recipes marked "V" are all-vegetable and can be used from Day 1 on. Baked Acorn Squash is a great recipe for beginners—all you have to do is put it in the oven!

You'll find that many of the recipes rely on similar ingredients and cooking techniques. These are important to master because they will enable you to adapt recipes you love to make them acceptable for the diet. To highlight the key facilitators:

1. **Plain, low-fat yogurt and low-fat buttermilk.** I know, you hate plain yogurt and buttermilk! Well, a lot of people think they do. But try cooking with them. I don't know what I would do without them. They are both great in salad dressings, soups, and to add a creamy texture to sauces. Try substituting either when a recipe calls for cream or sour cream. Both are very adaptable in cooking. But don't boil them—they separate. Add either just before serving. Use buttermilk when you want a more liquid cream sauce, yogurt when you want a thicker consistency. Yogurt is also a great topping for fruit desserts. Flavor it with cinnamon or a bit of vanilla or almond extract.
2. **Lemon juice.** Flavors seem to perk up around lemon. I use it in almost all my salad dressings and as a marinade for just about anything I broil. When a vegetable sauté looks dry, I squeeze in a bit of lemon. If a ratatouille needs some zip, it's lemon again. It's a great way to add a little liquid when you need it, without adding

oil or butter. Make sure you use pure lemon juice if you buy it in the supermarket, and not the reconstituted variety.

3. **Teriyaki sauce.** A little goes a long way. I mix it with lemon to make it milder. Teriyaki is like lemon in my opinion. It's great in salad dressings and as a marinade. It does contain sugar and sodium, but you'll be using such a small amount that it's negligible. You can also use soy sauce as an alternate flavor. It is very high in sodium, however. If you like it, remember to cut it with lemon.

4. **Water sautéing.** The combination of approximately ¼ cup water, ¼ cup wine, and sliced or chopped onion is a miracle for sautéing. Somehow, the onion gets syrupy, which gives the dish a thickness that's desirable. Just don't use too much liquid, keep the proportions equal, and you'll be fine. Once you master the technique, you'll wonder why anyone would waste calories on sautéing with oil, which has 120 calories a tablespoon! You can adapt many of your favorite recipes to make them acceptable on the program by using this technique.

   Incidentally, when you are really comfortable with water sautéing, you can try browning things by letting all the liquid in the pan evaporate when you start your onion base. It's best to do this in a nonstick pan, but it also works in a stainless steel or enamel one.

   The bottom of the pan will begin to get brown. When you add a bit more liquid it will boil up rapidly and brown the onions. Once the onions are nicely browned, you can add a little more wine and then "brown" whatever else you're cooking. This can make for a messy cleanup job, depending on your pan, but it's worth it—and it works!

5. **Marinating and broiling.** You won't find many chicken and fish recipes in this chapter. Instead, I've

given you prototype recipes (i.e. Tuna Stuffed Potato, p. 172, and Chicken Mushroom Risotto, p. 176) that you can master and adapt. You can make an endless variety of easy chicken and fish recipes by marinating and broiling (see Herb-Broiled Scallops, p. 174, as an example). Spicy mustard is a wonderful marinade for poultry or fish. Add garlic to the mustard to make it zippier. As suggested in the Transition chapter, Teriyaki or soy and lemon juice, or just fresh lemon and lime juice, also make easy, instant marinades. Wine and tarragon are a good combination. For inspiration, read over your favorite recipes. Use any marinade suggested, but omit the oil. When in doubt, add lemon juice or wine.

6. **Garlic.** I use garlic liberally, in lots of recipes. I generally suggest using a more modest amount in recipes than I actually use myself. So if you're a garlic lover, feel free to up the quantities.

   I recommend fresh garlic for use in recipes. If you want a more convenient form, I'd suggest you look for the jars of crushed garlic that can now be found in the refrigerator or spice cases of supermarkets. Look for brands that contain no oil, and buy only fresh, not reconstituted, crushed garlic. Never use powdered garlic, or garlic salt. The flavor's not even in the same ball park as fresh, or the new, bottled, crushed, fresh kind. If you use a lot of raw garlic you might want to munch on parsley after eating. Some people swear it cleans your breath.

7. **Cooking extra.** One of the ways to make cooking easy is to plan ahead and cook extra helpings. When I cook brown rice, I make enough for eight and freeze it in one-cup plastic containers. I make huge quantities of soup, freeze containers of it, and add all my leftover vegetables to the soup in my refrigerator so it takes on a variety of new flavors. (You can add anything to soup:

leftover salad, the lettuce leaves you'd usually discard,
anything that doesn't have yogurt or milk in it.) I even
bake potatoes ahead of time and slice them in half to
reheat, or stuff. I also save bits of one recipe to serve
as the base for another. Some leftover Vegetable Sauté
can become a pasta sauce by adding a bit of steamed
broccoli. Get the idea?

8. **Freezing.** As I just mentioned, cooking ahead and
freezing is a great way to make life easy. I also freeze
many prepared foods so that I can enjoy greater variety.
For example, I buy several kinds of fresh whole-grain
breads, have them presliced, and freeze them. Then I
toast them one slice at a time as needed. I also preslice
my bagels so that I can freeze and toast them a half at
a time. Freezing fruit is a great idea for dessert. Frozen
bananas, melon, and pineapple all work well. They get
a consistency that resembles sherbet when they defrost
for a few minutes. You can mix in yogurt if you like.
Frozen grapes make a wonderful addition to fruit
salads.

SOUPS

BASIC VEGETABLE STOCK (V)

*3–4 stalks celery, with leaves,
  chopped*
4–5 large carrots, chopped
2–3 parsnips, cut in half
2 onions, quartered
*One bunch fresh broccoli,
  chopped, including stalks
  and stems*

½ cup chopped parsley
5–6 garlic cloves, pressed
2–3 bay leaves
1 tablespoon thyme
1 tablespoon basil
3 quarts water
Salt to taste, if desired

Place all ingredients in a large kettle. Bring to boil, lower heat, and simmer for 2 hours. Strain stock through a colander to remove vegetable pieces. This makes a perfect base for the soup recipes that follow. When you clean vegetables for cooking, be sure to save the scraps you'd normally throw out to use for stock (as indicated above with broccoli stems). Makes about 2 quarts. Serves 8.

Nutritional information for one serving:

Calories:	*12*
Protein:	*0 grams*
Carbohydrate:	*4 grams*
Fat:	*0 gram*

HEARTY CABBAGE SOUP (V)

1 head cabbage, hard stem removed, sliced thin

6 cups water, defatted beef broth (see Note), or vegetable stock

1 28-ounce can whole tomatoes, packed in puree

1 large sweet onion, sliced

¼ cup red wine vinegar

2–3 large carrots, shredded (optional)

This is really simple. Place all ingredients in a large kettle. Bring to a boil. Simmer partially covered for 1–2 hours, until cabbage is tender. That's all there is to it. You can add carrots if you like. I add leftover vegetables as I have them, so that this usually starts out as a cabbage soup and ends up more like a cabbage mélange by the end of the week. Once you're on Stabilization, you can add canned kidney, lima, or other beans to make this soup a delicious, one-dish meal. Add them as you heat individual servings, or you'll make the soup too calorie-laden for snacking. Serves 6.

Note: The best way to "defat" chicken or beef broth is to leave it in the refrigerator overnight. The fat will harden on

top and you can remove it easily. If you use canned broth and
don't have time to do this, just skim off the visible fat when
you open the can.

Nutritional information for one serving:	
Calories:	93
Protein:	3 grams
Carbohydrate:	19 grams
Fat:	1 gram

BASIC VEGETABLE SOUP (V)

3–4 stalks celery, chopped
1 large Bermuda onion,
  chopped
1–2 cloves garlic, minced
2 carrots, grated
3 cups coarsely chopped
  zucchini, broccoli, or
  cauliflower (or a
  combination)

1 16-ounce can whole
  tomatoes, packed in puree
Seasonings to taste (thyme,
  marjoram, basil, or oregano
  —about ½ teaspoon)
6 cups liquid (use vegetable
  stock, water, tomato juice,
  and/or defatted beef or
  chicken broth, or a
  combination)

You can't make a mistake with vegetable soup. Any combination of vegetables will work. The liquid should just cover the
cut-up vegetables. Simmer all the ingredients 1½ hours, or
longer. Season to taste. I prefer to go light on the seasonings
and I vary them from batch to batch. If you want, you can
purée in a blender to thicken. Add leftover vegetables as you
have them. I even add leftover salad, as long as there's no
yogurt in the dressing. Mustard and vinegar just make the
soup tangy.

You never need to waste vegetables if you've got a soup
in the refrigerator. Whatever doesn't get eaten goes into it.
Don't discard the outer, tough leaves of a head of lettuce;

throw them in the soup! Remember that after Transition is completed, any beans you put in your soup help make it a main meal. Don't forget to add the beans with each serving, so that you can continue to eat the soup as a snack whenever you want. Serves 6–8. (Nutritional information based on 7 servings.)

Nutritional information for one serving:	
Calories:	75
Protein:	3 grams
Carbohydrate:	15 grams
Fat:	0 gram

ZUCCHINI SOUP* (V)

6 small to medium zucchini, peeled and coarsely cut (reserve ½ cup, cut in thin strips, for garnish)
2 large onions, chopped

½ teaspoon curry powder
4 cups defatted chicken broth or vegetable stock
Dill or chives for garnish

Zucchini Soup is delicious hot or cold. It's inexpensive and takes only a few minutes to prepare. Place chopped zucchini and onion in saucepan. Sprinkle with curry powder and stir to coat pieces. Add broth. Bring to boil. Cover and simmer 40–45 minutes. Spoon mixture into blender or food processor and purée. Garnish with reserved zucchini strips. Chill if desired. Serve sprinkled with dill or chopped chives. Serves 6.

Note: If you like your food on the spicy side, you can add a bit more curry powder. Be careful, though—it can get hot!

Optional: Add 1 tablespoon yogurt per serving.

*Substitute yellow squash if desired.

Nutritional information
for one serving:
Calories: 56
Protein: 2 grams
Carbohydrate: 12 grams
Fat: 0 grams

CARROT AND TURNIP SOUP (V)

*2–3 pounds carrots, cut in
bite-size pieces
1–2 pounds large parsnips, cut
in bite-size pieces
1–2 large yellow turnips
(rutabaga), cut in bite-size*

*pieces
6–8 cups defatted chicken
stock, vegetable stock, or
water (or a mixture)
Dash nutmeg*

This is a slightly sweet soup. It's great as a different taste during Transition. A mug of it can satisfy a sweet craving very successfully before you're allowed fruit. All you do is simmer all ingredients 1¼–2 hours. Purée in blender if desired. Serves 8.

Optional: Add 1 tablespoon yogurt per serving.

Nutritional information
for one serving:
Calories: 125
Protein: 2 grams
Carbohydrate: 28 grams
Fat: 0 grams

GAZPACHO (V)

*2 cucumbers, finely chopped
1 medium onion, finely
chopped*

*1 green pepper, seeded and
chopped
4 large ripe tomatoes, chopped*

1–2 cloves garlic, finely minced
1 cup tomato juice
2 tablespoons wine vinegar

⅛ teaspoon cayenne pepper
(optional)

GARNISH:
1 cucumber, seeded, peeled,
and diced

1 green pepper, seeded and
diced
2 scallions, finely sliced

Process vegetables and garlic in a blender or food processor. Blend with tomato juice and vinegar. Stir well. Chill. Add garnish just before serving. Serves 4–6. (Nutritional information based on 5 servings.)

Nutritional information for one serving:	
Calories:	87
Protein:	5 grams
Carbohydrate:	20 grams
Fat:	0 grams

BASIC GREEN SOUP

½ cup parsley
2 heads leafy green lettuce
(Boston, romaine, escarole,
etc.)
2 cups defatted chicken stock or
vegetable stock

1 small can peas, undrained
Pinch of salt and freshly
ground pepper

Green soups are great. Any greens will work in this. Feel free to add broccoli and spinach as well. Tear up the greens into bite-size pieces. Simmer all ingredients 20 minutes, or longer if you use a green like broccoli. Purée in a blender or food processor, if desired. Season to taste.

Although this soup is all-vegetable, it isn't permitted on Transition because of the peas. You can make it without them but even one small can does add a rich flavor. Serves 4.

Nutritional information
for one serving:
Calories: 51
Protein: 2 grams
Carbohydrate: 10 grams
Fat: 0 gram

COOL CUCUMBER BUTTER-MILK SOUP

3 cucumbers, peeled, seeded, and chopped
4 cups low-fat buttermilk
1 tablespoon lemon juice

1 tablespoon fresh dill (1 teaspoon dried)
1 tablespoon fresh mint (1 teaspoon dried), for garnish

Here's a perfect summer cooler that's a great way to start a light meal. Place all ingredients in a blender. Process until smooth. Garnish with mint leaves.

Note: Just a word about buttermilk. I use it to vary the flavor of any soup. Simply add a small amount to the portion that you're serving. It will give it a rich, creamy flavor. Buttermilk turns a vegetable soup into a cream of vegetable soup. It's also an excellent alternative to yogurt for making sauces creamy. It's not quite as thick, and is slightly less tart. Be sure to use only the low-fat variety.

If you can't find low-fat or skim buttermilk, use skim milk with 1 tablespoon vinegar added per 8 ounces. Serves 4.

Nutritional information
for one serving:
Calories: 114

Protein:	18 grams
Carbohydrate:	10 grams
Fat:	0 gram

ITALIAN CLAM SOUP

4 dozen littleneck clams
1 cup chopped onion
4–6 cloves garlic, finely minced
1¼ cup dry white wine
2¼ cup water
Salt and freshly ground black pepper to taste
4 anchovy fillets, drained and chopped (omit if on a salt-restricted diet)

1 teaspoon dried basil
3 tablespoons finely chopped fresh parsley
1 teaspoon oregano (slightly more if you've omitted the anchovies)
1 teaspoon crushed fennel seeds
1 six-ounce can tomato paste

I can't remember where I found this recipe, but I've used my variation of it, and loved it, for years. Just because the ingredients list is long doesn't mean it's difficult. It's a very easy recipe that's great for company. Scrub the clams well to remove all sand. Using a large pot with a tight-fitting cover, sauté the onion and garlic in ¼ cup of the water and ¼ cup of the wine until onion is translucent, about 5 minutes. Add the anchovies, basil, parsley, oregano, and fennel. Simmer 5 minutes. Add the tomato paste and the remaining wine and water. Stir. Simmer for 5 minutes more, then add the clams. Cover and boil, shaking the pot to stir up the clams, for 5–10 minutes, stirring occasionally, until all the clams open. Add salt and pepper, if needed.

Serve in hot bowls. You can float a piece of garlic toast in each bowl. (This can be made without oil by slicing an Italian or French bread into rounds, and allowing it to stand for several hours. Then rub each piece with a cut clove of garlic,

or pressed garlic, before toasting.) If you prefer, you can add
2 cups of cooked shells or macaroni, instead. Serves 4.

*Nutritional information
for one serving:*
Calories:	*274*
Protein:	*27 grams*
Carbohydrate:	*18 grams*
Fat:	*6 grams*

SALADS

STRING BEAN AND CARROT SALAD (V)

2 pounds string beans   *2 sweet red peppers (optional)*
4 medium carrots

The colors in this salad are beautiful, and the crunch of
crisply cooked beans and carrots makes it very satisfying.
Trim ends from beans. Scrape carrots and cut them into
thirds and then strips. Core and seed peppers and cut them
into thin strips. Steam beans and carrots briefly, about 5–7
minutes. Don't overcook! Leave red peppers raw. Combine
vegetables. Toss with Creamy Vinaigrette (see page 154),
and chill. Basil is a wonderful herb to add to the dressing
before tossing. And, after you're on Stabilization, a tablespoon of crumbled feta cheese is another delicious variation.
Serves 4.

*Nutritional information
for one serving:*
Calories:	*108*
Protein:	*6 grams*
Carbohydrate:	*24 grams*
Fat:	*0 grams*

SIMPLE CABBAGE SLAW (V)

1 head cabbage, shredded   *One small onion, sliced very*
2 carrots, shredded   *thin (optional)*

Go ahead and eat a lot of this one without a second thought. Simply combine ingredients and mix with Zesty Horseradish Dressing (see page 155). Serves 6.

Nutritional information	
for one serving:	
Calories:	*38*
Protein:	*2 gram*
Carbohydrate:	*9 grams*
Fat:	*0 grams*

SPINACH SALAD (V)

1 bunch fresh spinach   *1 red pepper, cut in thin*
1 hard-cooked egg white   *strips, or 1 Spanish onion,*
                                  cut in thin rings (optional)

The red pepper really perks up the spinach. Of course, I think red pepper perks up just about everything. Combine and toss with Creamy Vinaigrette (see page 154). Again, after you're on Stabilization, a tablespoon of crumbled feta or grated Parmesan makes a nice addition. Serves 2. (Nutritional information does not include feta or Parmesan cheese.)

Nutritional information	
for one serving:	
Calories:	*46*
Protein:	*4 grams*
Carbohydrate:	*8 grams*
Fat:	*1 gram*

CUCUMBER SALAD

6 large cucumbers, peeled and
  sliced very thin
4–6 sprigs fresh dill (1–2
  teaspoons dried)

1–1½ cups white vinegar, or
  as needed
1–2 teaspoons apple juice
  concentrate
Pinch salt

Notice the apple juice concentrate. I don't drink fruit juice,
but I do use fruit juice concentrate to sweeten. It is caloric,
but a little goes a long way. After you're on Personalization,
a pinch of sugar works well in this recipe. By then, you might
prefer the apple juice, however. Store the unused concentrate in the freezer but be sure to remove it from the original
container as oxidation can dangerously affect the contents of
any opened can. Use a plastic container or freezer bag.

To make the salad, just combine cucumbers and dill with
enough vinegar to barely cover, then add the apple juice
concentrate. Add a pinch of salt and chill before serving.
Serves 4–6. (Nutritional information based on 5 servings.)

Nutritional information for one serving:	
Calories:	53
Protein:	3 grams
Carbohydrate:	9 grams
Fat:	0 grams

CARROT SALAD

2–3 large carrots, shredded
Juice of ½ lemon
1 tablespoon Pommery or
  grainy mustard

2 tablespoons red wine or
  balsamic vinegar

This is a great salad to use as garnish for other dishes because
the color provides an attractive contrast. It's also delicious

with raw vegetables in a pita pocket, and it makes an appealing topping for potatoes. Simply mix all the ingredients in a medium-size bowl. Add additional mustard and/or vinegar to taste. Serves 2.

Nutritional information for one serving:
Calories: 74
Protein: 2 grams
Carbohydrate: 17 grams
Fat: 0 grams

CAESAR POTATO SALAD

3 pounds red boiling potatoes
1 medium bunch of parsley, chopped
2-3 scallions, chopped
4 tablespoons Parmesan cheese, grated

Juice of half a lemon
1 clove garlic
¼ cup Teriyaki sauce
Black pepper
¾ cup white vinegar
1 egg white

Here's a potato salad that can rival any you've ever tasted. In boiling water, cook potatoes in their skins, chill, cut in quarters, and set aside. In food processor or blender, purée egg white and garlic. Add vinegar, Teriyaki sauce, Parmesan cheese and lemon. Gently toss dressing in with potatoes along with scallions and parsley. Season to taste with pepper. Serves 4-6. (Nutritional information based on 5 servings.)

Nutritional information for one serving:
Calories: 153
Protein: 6 grams
Carbohydrate: 30 grams
Fat: 1 gram

DRESSINGS

Note: Egg whites can be added to any of the salad dressings below to extend them, make them less tart, or give them a thicker consistency.

CREAMY VINAIGRETTE (V)

*1 tablespoon dijon, Pommery,
or other hot or grainy
mustard
½ cup plain, low-fat yogurt*

*Juice of ½ lemon
2 tablespoons wine vinegar
(rice, red, or white)
Black pepper*

Shake ingredients in a covered jar or mix in a blender. I make endless variations on this basic dressing. By changing the mustard and vinegar I use, I can vary the flavor so that I'm never tired of it. The proportions are approximate. I purposely emphasize the mustard sometimes, and the vinegar at others. Experiment with vinegars. Japanese rice wine vinegar is slightly sweet. Traditional red or white wine vinegar is more classic in taste. Balsamic vinegar is stronger, and delicious. You can also use tomato or vegetable juice to vary the flavor. Makes approximately ¾ cup.

Note: 2 tablespoons dressing equals 1 tablespoon yogurt allotment.

Nutritional information for one tablespoon:	
Calories:	6
Protein:	*0 grams*
Carbohydrate:	*1 gram*
Fat:	*0 grams*

ZESTY HORSERADISH
DRESSING (V)

½ cup plain, low-fat yogurt
2 tablespoons plain vinegar
2 tablespoons horseradish

1 teaspoon finely chopped
  scallion or shallot
Salt and pepper

Shake ingredients in a jar or whir in a blender. This is great on the Cabbage Slaw (see page 151). It's also a good dressing for cold chicken or fish. Makes approximately ¾ cup.

Note: 1½ tablespoons dressing equals 1 tablespoon yogurt allotment.

Nutritional information for one tablespoon:	
Calories:	16
Protein:	0 grams
Carbohydrate:	4 grams
Fat:	0 grams

TOFU DRESSING

½-inch square fresh soybean
  custard (tofu)

¼ cup white, rice, or red wine
  vinegar

Mix in a blender or food processor and flavor with curry, mustard, basil, oregano, lemon, soy, or Teriyaki (use one at a time!). I'm not a big fan of tofu. In general, I find it's too bland for my taste. It makes a great base for salad dressing, however. If the Creamy Vinaigrette is too tart for you, this dressing might be preferable. It's just as versatile and it's easy to make. If it gets too tart, just add more tofu. Makes approximately 2 cups.

Nutritional information
for ⅓ cup:
Calories: 18
Protein: 2 grams
Carbohydrate: 1 gram
Fat: 1 gram

EASY MUSTARD DRESSING (V)

4 tablespoons grainy mustard   Juice of ½ lemon
   (Pommery or similar)   1–2 tablespoons wine vinegar

No time? Just squeeze some lemon and add a tablespoon of
vinegar to strong mustard. These quantities are approximate.
You can make more, shake the mixture in a covered jar, and
store it in your refrigerator. Makes approximately ¾ cup.

Nutritional information
for 1 tablespoon:
Calories: 8
Protein: 1 gram
Carbohydrate: 1 gram
Fat: 0 grams

ZIPPY MUSTARD DRESSING
PASTA SAUCE

4 tablespoons grainy mustard   1–2 cloves garlic, minced
   (Pommery or similar)   4 anchovy fillets, drained and
3 tablespoons lemon juice   mashed (optional)
2 tablespoons chopped scallion

Combine all ingredients in a jar, or mash together with a
mortar and pestle. This dressing is great on beets, asparagus,
and broccoli. It also makes a delicious cold pasta salad. Just
mix with bits of steamed vegetables and pasta, while the pasta

is warm. Serve at room temperature. Incidentally, I prefer more garlic and anchovies but was afraid to make it too overpowering for those who don't. If you're on a salt-restricted diet, omit the anchovies altogether. Use your judgment. Makes approximately ½ cup.

Nutritional information for ¾ recipe:	
Calories:	46
Protein:	4 grams
Carbohydrate:	4 grams
Fat:	3 grams

ORIENTAL DRESSING (V)

2 tablespoons Teriyaki sauce
2 tablespoons fresh lemon juice

Diced shallots or scallions (optional)

Mix Teriyaki sauce and lemon juice. What could be easier? Makes approximately ¼ cup.

Nutritional information for 1 tablespoon:	
Calories:	10
Protein:	0 grams
Carbohydrate:	2 grams
Fat:	0 grams

PUREED EGGPLANT DIP (V)

1 large eggplant
1–2 tablespoons chopped onion
1 clove pressed raw garlic or 3–4 cloves Baked Garlic (see page 158)

2–3 tablespoon red wine vinegar, preferably balsamic
Juice of ½ lemon
½ teaspoon oregano
Few drops Tabasco

Bake eggplant 1 hour at 350° F. Remove from oven and cool for one hour. Scrape out flesh. Mix hot eggplant with all other ingredients. Chill. Use as a dip for Steamed Vegetables (see page 159); it's also delicious with vegetables in a pita. And you can make a great cold pasta salad by tossing it with ziti and slivers of red pepper. Makes approximately 2–3 cups.

Nutritional information for ½ cup:	
Calories:	56
Protein:	*3 grams*
Carbohydrate:	*13 grams*
Fat:	*0 grams*

BAKED GARLIC (V)

1 large whole head of garlic

This isn't exactly a dressing or a dip. I'm not sure what it is, except that it's delicious. Remove the outer casing from a whole head of garlic (the larger the individual cloves, the better—if you can find "elephant" garlic, that's the best). Leave the head intact. Place on a double-strength square of aluminum foil and sprinkle with water. Seal the foil, making a tight packet. Bake in a 375° F oven for 1 hour. The garlic will be soft and mushy. You'll need to slit the cloves with a sharp paring knife to remove the soft, incredibly sweet (yes, sweet) garlic inside. I use Baked Garlic as a spread on steamed and raw vegetables, in mashed potatoes, in place of raw garlic in the Puréed Eggplant Dip above, spread on crackers to complement a salad, and just plain, straight from the clove, as a healthful, low-calorie indulgence.

*Nutritional information
for one head of garlic:*
Calories: 40
Protein: 2 grams
Carbohydrate: 9 grams
Fat: 0 grams

HOT VEGETABLES, MAIN DISHES, AND SAUCES

STEAMED VEGETABLES (V)

Steaming is the ideal method for cooking vegetables. It's the most nutritious and aesthetically pleasing. If you aren't a vegetable lover now, a $5 steaming basket may well change your mind.

The basic method is simple. Just place an inch or two of water in a saucepan. Clean and cut vegetables attractively. Steam briefly, so color is bright and texture remains firm, usually 5–7 minutes (brussels sprouts take longer, 20 minutes or so). Select vegetables of different colors. Beans, carrots, onions, turnips, leeks, broccoli, cabbage, and cauliflower all work well. Serve with a salad dressing as a dip, or sprinkle with a dash of lemon, Teriyaki, or soy sauce.

BAKED ACORN SQUASH (V)

1 acorn squash   *Lemon juice*

Preheat oven to 375° F. Use a fork to poke a few holes in the skin of the squash. Place on aluminum foil and bake one hour. Slice in half and remove the seeds. Sprinkle with lemon juice or any permitted dressing.

The squash can be stored in your refrigerator and reheated as you want it. I remove the seeds, sprinkle with lemon juice, and wrap each half separately. It's good cold, so you can take it along for lunch, or a snack, during Transition.

Note: You can prepare butternut and spaghetti squash the same way. When you serve spaghetti squash, turn it upside down after you remove the seeds and scrape the strands out with a fork. Serve it with Easy Tomato Sauce (see page 169).

Nutritional information for ½ squash:	
Calories:	100
Protein:	3 grams
Carbohydrate:	0 grams
Fat:	0 grams

RATATOUILLE (V)

1 Bermuda onion, thinly sliced	1 16-ounce can whole tomatoes, packed in purée
⅓ cup water	
⅓ cup wine	2 cloves garlic, minced
1 eggplant, cut in 1-inch cubes (don't peel it!)	½ teaspoon oregano
	½ teaspoon basil
1 green pepper, sliced in strips	¼ teaspoon ground pepper
1 red pepper, sliced in strips	Juice of ½ lemon
2–3 zucchini, sliced in ½-inch rounds	Salt to taste, if desired

Ratatouille is one of my favorite recipes. It's great hot in the morning, with your baked potato. It's delicious cold, as a salad (add 1 tablespoon of vinegar per serving). I love it over pasta. And on Stabilization, you can mix it with ziti and crumbled feta cheese and bake it in a casserole.

To make it, just sauté the onion in water and wine until

wilted and the liquid is mostly absorbed. Add the eggplant and peppers and toss quickly. The eggplant will give up some water, so it's okay if it seems dry at first. If you need to, add a bit more water and wine. Add the zucchini and sauté a few minutes longer. Then add the rest of the ingredients and simmer, covered, for 30 minutes. Remove cover, turn up heat, and reduce sauce by letting it boil down, generally about 10 minutes. This will serve two as a main dish, more as a side or luncheon dish.

Nutritional information
for ½ recipe:
Calories: *123*
Protein: *6 grams*
Carbohydrate: *0 grams*
Fat: *0 grams*

CABBAGE SAUTÉ

1 small head cabbage,   *½ apple, grated*
  shredded   *1½ teaspoons caraway seed*
1 medium onion, thinly sliced   *Lemon juice*

Sauté all ingredients except caraway seed in ½ inch of water, vegetable stock, or defatted broth until wilted, 10–15 minutes. Sprinkle with lemon juice and caraway seed before serving. Serves 2–4. (Nutritional information based on one serving.)

Nutritional information
for one serving:
Calories: *72*
Protein: *3 grams*
Carbohydrate: 14 grams
Fat: *.5 grams*

STUFFED ONIONS

4 large Bermuda onions
⅓ cup dry white wine
½ pound fresh mushrooms, diced
½ teaspoon dried basil
1 package frozen chopped spinach, defrosted and squeezed dry

⅓ cup freshly made whole-wheat breadcrumbs
¼ cup grated Parmesan
¼ cup chopped parsley
Salt and pepper to taste, if desired
¾ cup defatted chicken stock or vegetable stock

This recipe looks difficult, but it's actually very easy to accomplish and more than worth the effort. It's a wonderful main dish vegetable entrée or use it as a side dish with a simple broiled chicken. Think of it in three stages: preparing the onion shells, preparing the stuffing, and baking and finishing. Preheat oven to 350° F.

To prepare the onions for stuffing: Trim off the root end, cut about ½ inch off the stem end, and peel away outer brown skin. Use a melon baller to scoop out the center portion of each onion. Leave about 3 layers (at least ¼-inch thick) for the shell. Chop the center portions of the onions: use ½ cup for the stuffing, and reserve the rest for another use. Place shells in a large pot, cover with water, and boil for 3–5 minutes. Do not overcook. Drain them upside down, on paper towels.

To prepare the stuffing: Use a large frying pan to sauté the chopped onions, in 2 tablespoons water and 2 tablespoons of the white wine, until they are translucent, about 5 minutes. Add the mushrooms and basil and cook another 3 minutes, until the mushrooms are just soft. Add the spinach, all but 1 tablespoon each of the breadcrumbs, Parmesan, and parsley, and one more tablespoon of the wine. Season with salt and pepper, if desired. Place the onion shells in a casserole just large enough to hold them, and stuff them, mounding the stuffing lightly on top. Pour the stock and remaining wine around them. Cover loosely with foil and bake for 1 hour at 350° F.

To finish the onions: Uncover the casserole, increase the oven temperature to 425° F, and sprinkle the reserved 1 tablespoon of breadcrumbs, Parmesan, and chopped parsley evenly over the tops. Return to oven for 15 minutes. Transfer the onions to a serving platter. Boil the cooking liquid in a small saucepan until it's reduced to about ⅓ cup. Pour over onions and serve. Serves 4.

Nutritional information	
for one serving:	
Calories:	*120*
Protein:	*7 grams*
Carbohydrate:	*16 grams*
Fat:	*3 grams*

BAKED EGGPLANT (V)

1 eggplant

I find eggplant to be just about the most satisfying vegetable there is. When you want something solid, especially during the first three days on Transition, think eggplant. Acorn and butternut squash are almost as good, but not as versatile.

Here's a no-frills way to bake eggplant. Halve the eggplant, lengthwise. Score across the fleshy top several times. Rub with a cut clove of garlic or, if you're a garlic fiend like I am, press a clove of garlic and spread it across the top. Sprinkle with lemon juice and pepper and bake, scored side up, for 25 minutes in a 425° F oven. You can top with Easy Tomato Sauce (see page 169), or serve it with stewed tomatoes. Serves 2.

*Nutritional information
for one serving:*
Calories: 86
Protein: 4 grams
Carbohydrate: 18 grams
Fat: 1 gram

BROILED EGGPLANT (V)

1 eggplant

This takes more effort than Baked Eggplant, but it's worth it. Slice the eggplant in 1-inch-thick rounds. Rub slices with cut clove of garlic or bits of pressed garlic, if desired. Place on a cookie sheet and broil about 7 minutes on each side. Watch carefully, it can burn easily. Again, a tomato sauce is great on this. The Easy Tomato Sauce (see page 169) or Greek Tomato Sauce (see page 169) both work well. Omit the feta cheese until you've completed Transition. Serves 2.

*Nutritional information
for one serving:*
Calories: 86
Protein: 4 grams
Carbohydrate: 18 grams
Fat: 1 gram

EGGPLANT AND RICE CASSEROLE

2 large, firm eggplants (about 2 pounds total weight)
¼ cup tomato juice (from the canned tomatoes, below)
¼ cup white wine

3 cups minced onion
1 green pepper, cut into 1-inch cubes
2 cloves garlic, minced
½ teaspoon dried thyme

1 bay leaf
1 16-ounce can whole
  tomatoes, drained and
  chopped
1 cup uncooked brown rice

3 ½ cups defatted chicken
  stock or vegetable stock
Salt and freshly ground
  pepper, to taste
½ cup grated Parmesan cheese

This is a very satisfying, one-dish dinner. Preheat oven to
375° F. Trim the ends off the eggplant, slice, and cut into
1-inch cubes. Sauté the cubes in the tomato juice and wine
until just soft. Add the onion, green pepper, garlic, thyme,
and bay leaf. Simmer, stirring, for a few minutes. Add the
tomatoes and continue cooking 5–10 minutes, until the liquid is absorbed. The ingredients must be thick, so continue
to cook if too liquidy. Stir in the rice and stock and season
with salt and pepper, if desired. Spoon into a nonstick baking
dish. Sprinkle with grated cheese and bake, uncovered, for
45 minutes, until all the stock is absorbed and the rice is
tender. If the rice needs to cook longer, just turn off the oven
and let it sit for 10 minutes. To vary this dish, you can add
a 1-pound can of white cannelini beans when you add the
rice. It's more caloric, but it contains an excellent source of
low-fat protein. Serves 8.

Nutritional information
for one serving:
Calories: 198
Protein: 7 grams
Carbohydrate: 36 grams
Fat: 3 grams

BASIC VEGETABLE SAUTÉ (V)

1 large onion, thinly sliced
2 cloves garlic, minced
¼ cup white wine
¼ cup water

2 sweet red peppers, thinly
  sliced
¾ pound mushrooms
Salt and pepper to taste

¼ cup dry sherry (optional)   *1–2 tablespoons plain, low-fat
                                        yogurt with ⅛ teaspoon
                                        nutmeg (optional)*

If I had to choose one thing to live on, it might be Vegetable
Sauté over pasta. Any and all combinations work. During the
first three days of Transition, you can just eat the Sauté plain.
I use it as a side vegetable dish with fish all the time. Still,
using the method in this recipe, you can have a different
vegetable every night over pasta. I ask you, is this any way
to diet? Here's how to make it:

Sauté the onion and garlic in white wine and water 5–10
minutes, until wilted. Add red pepper and sauté 5 minutes
more. Add the mushrooms. Sauté 10 minutes, until the
mushrooms "give up" their juice. Reduce liquid over high
heat by letting it boil down. You may need to remove some
liquid. Save it to sauté another vegetable. If desired, add salt
and pepper and a bit of sherry at the end. Boil briefly. Stir
in 1 or 2 tablespoons of yogurt, flavored with ⅛ teaspoon
nutmeg, if desired once it's slightly cooled. Serves 2–4.

Note: This recipe can be adapted to a number of vegetables. Always begin with an onion in wine and water. It gives
the sauté a syrupy, thick base. Other vegetables that work
well are green peppers, scallions, leeks, eggplant, and
tomatoes. If you use broccoli or cauliflower you might want
to cover the pan for 3–5 minutes at the end to let them steam
to their bright, crispy best.

---

*Nutritional information
for ½ recipe:*

Calories:	*191*
Protein:	*9 grams*
Carbohydrate:	*28 grams*
Fat:	*0 grams*

VEGETABLE-BASED SPAGHETTI SAUCE

Use the method for Basic Vegetable Sauté. Don't reduce the sauce too far. Reserve yogurt. Cook spaghetti, drain. Mix the hot spaghetti with yogurt (1 tablespoon per serving). Spoon hot vegetable sauté over spaghetti and yogurt and serve. Once you're on Stabilization you can adopt this recipe to include 1 tablespoon per serving of a mild chevre (goat cheese) like Montrachet. Toss the hot spaghetti with the sauce and cheese before serving. It's incredibly delicious.

If you like, you can purée the sauce before serving for a thick, rich texture. You can purée the following sauces, as well, which seems to give them a different taste as well as appearance.

Note: Serving size of spaghetti is 1 cup, cooked.

MUSHROOM SPAGHETTI SAUCE

1 large Bermuda onion, thinly sliced
2–3 cloves garlic, minced
Dash nutmeg
Salt and pepper
¼ cup water
¼ cup sherry

1–2 pounds fresh mushrooms, thickly sliced
2 tablespoons chopped parsley
2 tablespoons plain, low-fat yogurt (optional)
½ pound spaghetti

This is really just a more specific version of the Basic Vegetable Sauté described above. It's so easy, though, that I wanted to be sure to highlight it. Sauté the onion, garlic, nutmeg, salt, and pepper in the water and sherry until wilted. Wait until you start the spaghetti to add the mushrooms to the onions. Sauté for about 8 minutes, until they give up their liquid, and are just tender. Drain the spaghetti and then toss with the mushroom sauce, over the heat, before serving. If you want it creamier, add 1 tablespoon yogurt to each serving, once it's off the heat. Serve with sprinkled parsley.

After Transition, you can substitute 1 tablespoon crumbled goat cheese (like Montrachet) or feta per serving, for the yogurt. Be sure to add cheese after the sauce is off the heat. On Stabilization, you might want to add a small can of baby peas, drained, to the sauce just before you take it off the heat. Serves 2–4.

Nutritional information for ⅓ recipe:

Calories:	*101*
Protein:	*6 grams*
Carbohydrate:	*14 grams*
Fat:	*1 gram*

SPAGHETTI AND BROCCOLI

1 medium onion, chopped
2 cloves garlic, minced
2 teaspoons dried basil (4 tablespoons fresh)
¼ cup water
¼ cup wine

1 bunch fresh broccoli, chopped in small flowerettes and stem slices
½ pound spaghetti
2 tablespoons plain, low-fat yogurt (optional)

Here's another vegetable pasta sauce to help you get the idea. Sauté the onion, garlic, and basil in the water and wine. Steam the broccoli briefly, about 5–7 minutes, in the pot in which you'll cook your spaghetti. Add the steamed broccoli to the onion. Add to the base of broccoli water for your spaghetti water. You can toss the cooked spaghetti with yogurt before you top with sauce. Serve with grated Parmesan, if desired, 1 tablespoon per person. Serves 2–4.

*Nutritional information
for ⅓ recipe:*
Calories: 73
Protein: 6 grams
Carbohydrate: 11 grams
Fat: 1 gram

EASY TOMATO SAUCE (V)

1 medium onion, chopped
1–2 cloves garlic, pressed
1 16-ounce can whole
  tomatoes, packed in purée

Salt and pepper, basil, or
  oregano to taste

This sauce tastes so much fresher than canned tomato sauces
that it's worth the twenty minutes it takes to make it. Sauté
the onion and garlic in a little of the tomato juice from the
can. When onion and garlic are soft, add the tomatoes (you
can shop them first) and seasonings and simmer for 15 minutes. Serves 2.

*Nutritional information
for one serving:*
Calories: 53
Protein: 2 grams
Carbohydrate: 11 grams
Fat: 0 grams

GREEK ·TOMATO SAUCE

2 cloves garlic, chopped
¼ cup wine
1 28-ounce can Italian
  tomatoes
¼ cup bottled clam juice

1 teaspoon oregano
½ teaspoon dried hot red
  pepper flakes
2 tablespoons drained capers
2 ounces crumbled feta cheese

Sauté garlic in the wine for 3–5 minutes. Add the tomatoes and cook over a moderately high heat, until the liquid is reduced by about a third. Add the clam juice, seasonings, and capers. Simmer 10 minutes. This distinctive tomato sauce is great served with crumbled feta cheese over any thick white fish or shellfish. Just before fish is done, top with sauce and cheese, and run under broiler briefly, until bubbling. Serves 4.

Add 2 tablespoons vinegar to make a delicious dressing for a cold seafood salad. Or try a seafood risotto with this Greek-inspired sauce.

Note: Omit the cheese until Stabilization.

Nutritional information for one serving with cheese:		*Nutritional information for one serving without cheese:*	
Calories:	*103*	*Calories:*	*66*
Protein:	*5 grams*	*Protein:*	*3 grams*
Carbohydrate:	*12 grams*	*Carbohydrate:*	*12 grams*
Fat:	*4 grams*	*Fat:*	*0 grams*

ZESTY TOMATO SAUCE

1 large Bermuda onion
4–5 stalks celery
2–3 cloves garlic
4 flat anchovy fillets (more if you want it spicier and are not on a salt-restricted diet)
¼ cup water

¼ cup white or red wine
1 28-ounce can Italian tomatoes, packed in purée
3 tablespoons capers
½ teaspoon basil
Black pepper

Chop the onion, celery, and garlic very fine. You can use a food processor or blender. If they get "mushy," that's okay. Sauté them with the anchovy fillets in the water and wine over a high heat, until the liquid boils down and the consistency is thick. Add the tomatoes, capers, basil, and black pepper, and simmer for 20 minutes. Once you're on Personalization, or if you're cooking for guests, you can add a few chopped olives. I buy spicy Italian or Greek olives. Just a few, about six, are all you need. Add them with the other spices. Serves 4.

Note: Many people are squeamish about anchovies. Don't be in this recipe. They disintegrate in cooking, and you can't taste them as anchovies. They add a great flavor. If you need to watch your salt intake, you can omit them. If you do, substitute the juice of ½ lemon just before serving, and go a little heavier on the garlic, pepper, and basil.

Serve with Parmesan or romano cheese. Limit 1 tablespoon per person (not per serving!). If you like to keep portions small and take seconds, save some of your cheese for that extra serving.

Nutritional information for ½ cup:	
Calories:	56
Protein:	3 grams
Carbohydrate:	9 grams
Fat:	1 gram

SPAGHETTI WITH WHITE CLAM SAUCE

3 cloves or more garlic, minced
2 tablespoons chopped fresh parsley
3 scallions, minced
3 shallots, minced
1 teaspoon dried oregano

⅓ cup water
½ cup white wine
3–4 dozen clams, scrubbed and rinsed very well
1 pound spaghetti

This sauce is heavenly. You'll never miss the oil! Sauté garlic, parsley, scallions, shallots, and oregano in the water and wine for a few minutes in an uncovered large frying pan that has a tight-fitting lid. Raise the heat and boil down the liquid until it just covers the bottom of the pan. Add the clams. Cover. Keep on a high heat. Cook, stirring occasionally, for 5 minutes or so, until clams open. Remove the open clams (a set of tongs is the best utensil for this step) and scoop them out of their shells. Reserve the clams. Be sure not to remove the clam liquid when you take them out of the pot. Chop the clams. Add the spaghetti to boiling water and cook for 8 minutes (noodles should still be firm) while you allow the clam juice to boil down by about half. If it boils down too far, you can add more wine. Add the chopped clams. Toss with spaghetti. You might want to reserve a few of the clam shells, to garnish the plate. Serves 4–6.

Nutritional information for ¼ of recipe:

Calories:	*119*
Protein:	*15 grams*
Carbohydrate:	*4 grams*
Fat:	*4 grams*

TUNA-STUFFED POTATO

1 baked potato
1 3½-ounce can water-packed tuna
1 stalk celery, chopped
1 tablespoon chopped onion
1 tablespoon cottage cheese (1% fat)

2 tablespoons plain, low-fat yogurt
1½ tablespoons dijon or other mustard

Again, this is a prototype recipe. You can mix leftover vegetables with potatoes for stuffing just as easily as tuna. When you do, the recipe will be less caloric and contain less fat. It's a fast, easy solution to what to make for lunch or dinner. Just scoop out the potato meat and mix it with other ingredients. Stuff back into potato skins. Bake in a toaster oven at 375° F for 15–20 minutes, until crisp on top. Serves 1.

Note: You can substitute 1 tablespoon feta cheese for the cottage cheese after Transition, or omit cheese from the stuffing and sprinkle with 1 tablespoon grated Parmesan.

> *Nutritional information*
> *for 1 serving:*
> *Calories:* 355
> *Protein:* 37 grams
> *Carbohydrate:* 38 grams
> *Fat:* 4 grams

SCOOPED-OUT BAGEL

4 bagels, sliced
8 ounces low fat cottage cheese, pureed
2 tablespoons chopped scallion
2 tablespoons grated Parmesan cheese
Tomato slices (optional)

Scoop out the bready part of the bagels and reserve for bread crumbs. Mix the pureed cottage cheese, scallion, and Parmesan cheese. Fill bagel halves with mixture, top with tomatoes, heat in a toaster oven for 10 minutes at 350° F, and "top brown" briefly before serving. It's a great quick breakfast, lunch, or dinner. Serves 4.

> *Nutritional information*
> *for one serving:*
> *Calories:* 150
> *Protein:* 9 grams
> *Carbohydrate:* 19 grams
> *Fat:* 4 grams

SCALLOP KABOBS

8 ounces sea scallops
Juice of ½ lemon and ½ lime
Tabasco
1 large onion, cut into squares
1 green or red pepper, cut into
 squares

8 mushroom caps, whole
4 cherry tomatoes
1 small zucchini, sliced in
 thick rounds

This recipe looks gorgeous, and it tastes as good as it looks!
Figure on two skewers per person. I usually thread extra
vegetables on an additional skewer. Marinate scallops in
lemon, lime, and Tabasco. They will give up liquid. Thread
skewers, alternating scallops and vegetables. Baste with liquid. Broil a few minutes, turning once or twice, and basting.
Serves 2.

Nutritional information
for one serving:
Calories: 194
Protein: 28 grams
Carbohydrate: 15 grams
Fat: 2 grams

HERB-BROILED SCALLOPS

1 pound scallops
1 teaspoon dried basil
½ teaspoon dried rosemary

2 lemons, one thinly sliced, one
 cut in wedges
Tabasco to taste
¼ cup dry white wine

Use either bay or sea scallops (you may cut sea scallops in half
if you prefer). Place all ingredients except lemon wedges in
a bowl and cover. Refrigerate for at least 2 hours. Stir every
hour. Remove scallops from the marinade and place in one

layer in baking dish. Broil for 3–5 minutes per side. Turn once. Do not overcook the scallops or they will toughen. Serve with fresh lemon wedges. Serves 4.

Nutritional information for one serving:	
Calories:	140
Protein:	26 grams
Carbohydrate:	1 gram
Fat:	2 grams

SOLE WITH TOMATOES

2 tablespoons chopped onion
¾ cup white wine
4 small fillets of sole (flounder also works well)
¼ cup bottled clam juice

1 cup canned tomatoes, drained and chopped
½ teaspoon dried basil
2 tablespoons parsley, chopped
Salt and freshly ground black pepper to taste

Here's a nice change from simple broiled fish. Sauté the onion in ¼ cup of the wine, about 5 minutes. Arrange the fillets in the pan and pour the clam juice and remaining wine over them. Add the tomatoes, basil, and parsley, and simmer on low heat for about 5 minutes. Turn and cook an additional 5 minutes, until the fish flakes easily when poked with a fork. Remove the fish to a warm serving platter. Boil the sauce over a low flame until it is reduced by half, about 3 minutes. Add the salt and pepper, if needed. Pour over the fish and serve. Serves 4.

Nutritional information for one serving:	
Calories:	172
Protein:	18 grams

| Carbohydrate: | 6 grams |
| Fat: | 5 grams |

CHICKEN AND MUSHROOM RISOTTO

1 small onion, or several shallots, chopped
2 cloves garlic, minced
½ pound mushrooms (half minced, half thickly sliced)
¼ cup white wine
¼ cup water

6 ounces cooked white chicken meat
Salt and pepper
1 ¾ cup liquid (use sauté liquid plus water)
½ cup uncooked brown rice
2 tablespoons plain, low-fat yogurt

Use this recipe as a blueprint for risotto. You can substitute broccoli or asparagus for the chicken. When I do, I add ⅛ cup of Parmesan cheese at the end of the recipe, along with the yogurt. I also use dried mushrooms to give it extra flavor. You just soak them in hot water for 20 minutes or so. Use their liquid to cook the rice and add the mushrooms, chopped, to the chicken-mushroom mixture. Even with dried mushrooms, you'll need fresh ones for "body." It's true that with classic risotto, you add the liquid very slowly, letting the rice absorb it bit by bit. Depending on my mood, I sometimes go through the whole process. But this method works well and it's much less trouble.

Just sauté onion, garlic, and minced mushrooms in the wine and water for 10 minutes. Add sliced mushrooms and chicken and sauté over medium heat an additional 6–7 minutes. Remove the chicken-mushroom mixture with a slotted spoon. Pour remaining liquid into 2 cup measure. Fill measure with water to 1¾ cup line. Add to saucepan with ½ cup brown rice. Bring to a boil. Lower heat and simmer, covered, for 35 minutes. Stir in chicken-mushroom mixture and yogurt. Cover and lower heat. Let steam an additional 5–10 minutes, until rice is just firm. Serves 4.

Nutritional information for one serving:	
Calories:	200
Protein:	17 grams
Carbohydrate:	24 grams
Fat:	2 grams

DESSERTS

The best dessert is fresh fruit. I frequently broil bananas (see recipe on page 65), or bake apples, or freeze pineapple. When I think dessert, I think fruit. What happens most often when you play with "mock cheese cake" is that you end up with a yen for the real thing. I know that you can make an "apple crisp" with pita and stewed apples; however, I think it's best to eat your grains with your meals.

Consequently, I recommend that you concentrate on the endless possibilities inherent in fruit desserts. Serving a fruit salad (1 cup = 1 serving) of fresh ripe pineapple and whole strawberries with a sprinkling of seedless green grapes makes a beautiful ending for any meal. Ripe papaya with fresh blueberries or strawberries is equally appealing. In fact, I can't think of a combination that wouldn't be tempting. The secret to combining fruits is to contrast them in color and texture. One other hint is to sprinkle cut fruit with fresh lemon juice to preserve color.

Besides Broiled Banana, another delicious hot dessert is baked apple. Simply remove the core and place apple in a deep baking dish. Add a few inches of water and a squeeze of lemon juice to the baking dish. Bake uncovered in a 350° F oven for 1 hour. Fill the apple's cavity with 1 tablespoon of plain, low-fat yogurt and a dash of cinnamon in the last 5 minutes of baking.

As I said earlier, freezing fruit is another wonderful innovation. It's best to peel bananas and wrap them in clear plastic wrap before freezing. Grapes, pineapple chunks, cut-up melon, even mango will freeze well in plastic containers. Before serving, you can whip up the fruit in a food processor or blender to create a sherbet-like texture.

9

Nutritional Listings

Although *The Bloomingdale's Eat Healthy Diet* has been specifically designed to work without the need for counting calories, knowing the caloric content of foods will help correct any misconceptions you might have. What's more critical, however, is their fat, protein, and carbohydrate makeup.

The following tables use cups, ounces, pounds, or some other well-known unit as a measure. To ensure that there's no confusion, I've included the gram weights (g) for each food so that you have a consistent measure for comparison. Only the edible part of the item is included in the calorie and nutrient count.

If not stated, nutrient analyses of vegetables are for fresh, frozen, or canned. Fresh vegetables, followed by frozen, then canned, have the highest vitamin and mineral density. The heating process destroys some vitamins, and both vitamins and minerals leach out into the water of canned vegetables. Carbohydrate, protein, fat, and caloric content, however, are not affected.

Read over the tables and familiarize yourself with the nutritive values of a wide range of foods. The more informed you are, the better able you will be to make choices that will help you reach your goal.

The following tables have been compiled by N Squared Computing, a software company in Silverton, Oregon, with their software program, Nutritionist I. The sources for the listings are *Nutritive Value of American Foods in Common Units,* Agriculture Handbook No. 456, Agriculture Research Service, U.S. Department of Agriculture, Washington, D.C., 1975; Bowes and Church's *Food Values of Portions Commonly Used,* 13th edition, Jean A. T. Pennington and Helen Nichols Church, Harper & Row, New York, 1980; and product information from the consumer services divisions of various food companies. The tables have been reviewed and supplemented by Julie Bukar, R.D., Research Metabolic Dietician at the Metabolism Research Unit of St. Luke's-Roosevelt Hospital in New York City.

Note: The following abbreviations are used in the tables: cnd. = canned; enr. = enriched; evap. = evaporated; froz. = frozen; HR = home recipe; hydrog. = hydrogenated; imit. = imitation; L & F = lean and fat; oz. = ounce(s); reg. = regular; swt. = sweetened; tbs. = tablespoon(s); unswt. = unsweetened; veg. = vegetable.

BEVERAGES

Food	Amount	Weight (g)	Calories	Protein (g)	Carbohydrate (g)	Fat (g)
Alcoholic						
Beer, Budweiser	12 oz.	360	150	1.1	14.0	0.0
Daiquiri	1 cocktail glass (3½ oz.)	100	122	.1	5.2	0.0
Hard liquor: 80 proof	1½ oz. = 1 jigger	45	104	0.0	0.0	0.0
Hard liquor: 100 proof	1½ oz. = 1 jigger	45	133	0.0	0.0	0.0
Old-fashioned	4 oz.	100	180	0.0	3.5	0.0
Wine, California, red	1 glass (3½ oz.)	100	85	0.0	4.0	0.0
Wine, California, sauterne	1 glass (3½ oz.)	100	85	0.0	4.0	0.0
Wine, vermouth, sweet (Italian)	1 glass (3½ oz.)	100	167	0.0	12.0	0.0
Carbonated						
Cream soda	12 oz.	360	155	0.0	39.6	0.0
Ginger ale	12 oz.	360	136	0.0	33.8	0.0
Pepsi-Cola	12 oz.	360	156	0.0	39.4	0.0
Seven-Up	12 oz.	360	144	0.0	36.0	0.0
Miscellaneous						
Café Viennese, instant	1 cup	240	62	0.0	12.7	0.0

B E V E R A G E S (Continued)

Food	Amount	Weight (g)	Calories	Protein (g)	Carbohydrate (g)	Fat (g)
Coffee, instant	1 cup	240	2	0.0	1.2	0.0
Hawaiian Punch	1 cup	250	120	.1	29.3	trace
Tea, orange pekoe tea bag	1 cup	240	2	.1	.5	0.0

D A I R Y

Food	Amount	Weight (g)	Calories	Protein (g)	Carbohydrate (g)	Fat (g)
Cheese, blue	1 oz.	28	100	6.0	1.0	8.0
Cheese, Cheddar, cut pieces	1 oz.	28	115	7.0	0.0	9.0
Cheese, Cheddar, shredded	1 tbs.	7	28	2.0	0.0	2.0
Cheese, cottage (1% fat)	3 oz.	84	61	10.0	2.0	1.0
Cheese, cottage (2% fat)	3 oz.	84	76	12.0	3.0	1.0
Cheese, cottage (4.2% fat), large or small curd	3 oz.	84	90	12.0	2.0	4.0
Cheese, cottage, uncreamed (0.3% fat)	3 oz.	84	72	9.0	1.0	0.0
Cheese, cream	1 oz.	28	100	2.0	1.0	10.0
Cheese, Edam	1 oz.	28	87	7.7	1.1	5.7
Cheese, feta	1 oz.	28	74	4.0	1.1	6.0

DAIRY (Continued)

Food	Amount	Weight (g)	Calories	Protein (g)	Carbohydrate (g)	Fat (g)
Cheese, Gouda	1 oz.	28	100	7.0	.6	7.7
Cheese, Gruyere	1 oz.	28	115	8.1	.5	8.9
Cheese, Mozzarella (skim milk)	1 oz.	28	80	8.0	1.0	5.0
Cheese, Mozzarella (whole milk)	1 oz.	28	90	6.0	1.0	7.0
Cheese, Muenster	1 oz.	28	104	6.6	.3	8.5
Cheese, Parmesan, grated	1 tbs.	5	25	2.0	0.0	2.0
Cheese, Parmesan, grated	1 oz.	28	130	12.0	1.0	9.0
Cheese, processed American	1 oz.	28	105	6.0	0.0	9.0
Cheese, processed spread	1 oz.	28	82	5.0	2.0	6.0
Cheese, processed Swiss	1 oz.	28	95	7.0	1.0	7.0
Cheese, provolone	1 oz.	28	100	7.0	1.0	8.0
Cheese, ricotta (skim milk)	1 cup	246	340	28.0	13.0	19.0
Cheese, ricotta (whole milk)	1 cup	246	430	28.0	7.0	32.0
Cheese, romano	1 oz.	28	110	9.0	1.0	8.0
Cheese, Swiss, grated	1 tbs.	7	26	2.0	0.0	2.0
Cream, froz. imit., whipped topping	1 cup	75	240	1.0	17.0	19.0
Cream, froz. imit., whipped topping	1 tbs.	4	15	0.0	1.0	1.0
Cream, half-and-half (11.7% fat)	1 cup	242	315	7.0	10.0	28.0
Cream, half-and-half (11.7% fat)	1 tbs.	15	20	0.0	1.0	2.0

DAIRY (Continued)

Food	Amount	Weight (g)	Calories	Protein (g)	Carbohydrate (g)	Fat (g)
Cream, heavy whipping	1 cup	238	820	5.0	7.0	88.0
Cream, heavy whipping	1 tbs.	15	80	0.0	0.0	6.0
Cream, heavy, whipped topping (37.6% fat)	1 cup	119	419	3.0	4.0	45.0
Cream, heavy, whipped topping (37.6% fat)	1 tbs.	15	53	0.0	1.0	6.0
Cream, light (20.6% fat)	1 cup	240	506	7.0	10.0	50.0
Cream, light (20.6% fat)	1 tbs.	15	32	0.0	1.0	3.0
Cream, sour	1 cup	230	495	7.0	10.0	48.0
Cream, sour	1 tbs.	12	25	0.0	1.0	3.0
Custard, baked	1 cup	265	305	14.0	29.0	15.0
Ice cream, reg. (11% fat)	1 cup	133	270	5.0	32.0	14.0
Ice cream, rich (16% fat)	1 cup	148	350	4.0	32.0	24.0
Ice cream, soft froz. custard	1 cup	173	375	7.0	38.0	23.0
Ice milk, hard (4.3% fat)	1 cup	131	185	5.0	29.0	6.0
Milk (1% fat, no milk solids)	1 cup	244	100	8.0	12.0	3.0
Milk (2% fat, no milk solids)	1 cup	244	120	8.0	12.0	5.0
Milk, buttermilk (skim)	1 cup	245	88	9.0	10.0	0.0
Milk, buttermilk (whole)	1 cup	244	92	8.0	12.0	2.0

DAIRY (Continued)

Food	Amount	Weight (g)	Calories	Protein (g)	Carbohydrate (g)	Fat (g)
Milk, chocolate (commercial)	1 cup	250	210	8.0	26.0	8.0
Milk, condensed, swt. (cnd.)	1 cup	306	980	24.0	166.0	27.0
Milk, eggnog (commercial)	1 cup	254	340	10.0	34.0	19.0
Milk, nonfat (skim) (no milk solids)	1 cup	245	85	8.0	12.0	0.0
Milk, nonfat instant	1 cup	68	245	24.0	35.0	0.0
Milk, nonfat instant (envelope)	3.2 oz.	91	325	32.0	47.0	1.0
Milk shake, chocolate	10.6 oz.	300	355	9.0	63.0	8.0
Milk shake, vanilla	11 oz.	313	350	12.0	56.0	9.0
Milk, whole (3.3% fat)	1 cup	244	150	8.0	11.0	8.0
Milk, whole, evap., unswt. (cnd.)	1 cup	252	340	17.0	25.0	19.0
Pudding, chocolate (instant)	1 cup	260	325	8.0	63.0	7.0
Pudding, chocolate (mix with milk)	1 cup	260	320	9.0	59.0	8.0
Sherbet (2% fat)	½ gal.	1542	2160	17.0	469.0	31.0
Sherbet (2% fat)	1 cup	193	270	2.0	59.0	4.0
Tofu, frozen (non-dairy)	8 oz.	227	440	4.0	60.0	20.0
Yogurt, fruit* (low-fat milk)	8 oz.	227	230	10.0	42.0	3.0

*Fruit yogurts vary with brand and flavor. Check label for exact calorie content and nutrie breakdown.

DAIRY (Continued)

Food	Amount	Weight (g)	Calories	Protein (g)	Carbohydrate (g)	Fat (g)
Yogurt, plain (low-fat milk, with nonfat milk solids)	8 oz.	227	145	12.0	16.0	4.0
Yogurt, plain (nonfat, milk solids)	8 oz.	227	125	13.0	17.0	0.0
Yogurt, plain (whole)	8 oz.	227	140	7.0	11.0	8.0

EGGS AND OILS

Food	Amount	Weight (g)	Calories	Protein (g)	Carbohydrate (g)	Fat (g)
Butter, reg.	1 tbs.	14	100	0.0	0.0	12.0
Butter, whipped	1 tbs.	9	65	0.0	0.0	8.0
Cooking fat, veg.	1 cup	200	1770	0.0	0.0	200.0
Cooking fat, veg.	1 tbs.	13	110	0.0	0.0	13.0
Egg white, raw	1 large	33	15	3.0	0.0	0.0
Egg, whole, raw	1 large	50	80	6.0	1.0	6.0
Egg yolk, raw	1 large	17	65	3.0	0.0	6.0
Egg (fried in butter)	1 large	46	85	5.0	1.0	6.0
Egg (hard-boiled)	1 large	50	80	6.0	1.0	6.0
Egg (poached)	1 large	50	80	6.0	1.0	6.0
Egg (scrambled, milk and butter)	1 large	64	95	6.0	1.0	7.0
Lard	1 cup	205	1850	0.0	0.0	205.0
Lard	1 tbs.	13	115	0.0	0.0	13.0
Margarine, reg.	1 tbs.	14	100	0.0	0.0	12.0
Margarine, soft	1 tbs.	14	100	0.0	0.0	12.0
Margarine, whipped	1 tbs.	9	70	0.0	0.0	8.0
Oil, corn	1 cup	218	1925	0.0	0.0	218.0

EGGS AND OILS (Continued)

Food	Amount	Weight (g)	Calories	Protein (g)	Carbohydrate (g)	Fat (g)
Oil, corn	1 tbs.	14	120	0.0	0.0	14.0
Oil, olive	1 cup	216	1910	0.0	0.0	216.0
Oil, olive	1 tbs.	14	120	0.0	0.0	14.0
Oil, peanut	1 cup	216	1910	0.0	0.0	216.0
Oil, peanut	1 tbs.	14	120	0.0	0.0	14.0
Oil, safflower	1 cup	218	1925	0.0	0.0	218.0
Oil, safflower	1 tbs.	14	120	0.0	0.0	14.0
Oil, soybean (hydrog.)	1 cup	218	1925	0.0	0.0	218.0
Oil, soybean (hydrog.)	1 tbs.	14	120	0.0	0.0	14.0
Oil, soybean/ cottonseed	1 cup	218	1925	0.0	0.0	218.0
Oil, soybean/ cottonseed	1 tbs.	14	120	0.0	0.0	14.0
Salad dressing, blue cheese	1 tbs.	15	75	1.0	1.0	8.0
Salad dressing, French	1 tbs.	16	65	0.0	3.0	6.0
Salad dressing, Italian	1 tbs.	15	85	0.0	1.0	9.0
Salad dressing, mayonnaise	1 tbs.	14	100	0.0	0.0	11.0
Salad dressing, tartar	1 tbs.	14	75	0.0	1.0	8.0
Salad dressing, Thousand Island	1 tbs.	16	80	0.0	2.0	8.0

FAST FOOD

Food	Amount	Weight (g)	Calories	Protein (g)	Carbohydrate (g)	Fat (g)
Banana split, Dairy Queen	1	383	540	10.0	91.0	15.0
Burrito, Taco Bell (Bean)	1	166	343	11.0	48.0	12.0
Burrito, Taco Bell (Beef)	1	184	466	30.0	37.0	21.0
Cheeseburger, McDonald's	1	114	306	15.6	30.4	13.3
Chicken, Kentucky Fried (original recipe)	1 thigh	97	276	20.0	12.0	19.0
Chili con carne and beans, Wendy's	1 serving	250	250	22.0	23.0	7.0
Egg McMuffin, McDonald's	1	132	352	18.0	26.0	20.0
Fish Sandwich, Arthur Treacher's	1	156	440	16.4	44.0	19.2
French fries, Burger King (reg.)	1 serving	43	214	3.0	28.0	10.0
Hamburger, Burger King	1	90	252	14.0	29.0	9.0
Hamburger, Wendy's single	1	200	440	25.0	33.0	25.0
Pizza, Pizza Hut (cheese)	½ of 1 10-inch pizza (3 slices)	NA	450	25.0	54.0	15.0
Shake, Wendy's (chocolate)	1	250	390	8.0	55.0	15.0

FISH AND SEAFOOD

Food	Amount	Weight (g)	Calories	Protein (g)	Carbohydrate (g)	Fat (g)
Bluefish (broiled)	½ fish	122	192	32.0	0.0	6.3
Clams, raw (meat only)	3 oz.	85	65	11.0	2.0	1.0
Clams, solids and liquid (canned)	3 oz.	85	45	7.0	2.0	1.0
Cod (broiled)	3 oz.	85	144	24.0	0.0	2.0
Crabmeat, king (canned)	1 cup	135	135	24.0	1.0	3.0
Fish sticks, breaded	1 oz. stick	28	50	5.0	2.0	3.0
Haddock (broiled)	3 oz.	85	121	17.2	0.2	5.6
Halibut (broiled)	3 oz.	86	147	21.5	0.0	6.0
Herring (broiled)	3 oz.	85	217	20.8	0.0	14.2
Oysters, raw (meat only)	1 cup	240	160	20.0	8.0	4.0
Salmon (broiled or baked)	3 oz.	86	156	23.0	0.0	6.3
Salmon, pink (canned)	3 oz.	85	120	17.0	0.0	5.0
Sardines (canned in oil)	3 oz.	85	175	20.0	0.0	9.0
Shrimp (canned)	3 oz.	85	100	21.0	1.0	1.0
Snails, raw	3 oz.	85	77	13.8	1.7	1.2
Sole (baked)	3 oz.	85	121	17.2	0.2	5.6
Sturgeon (steamed)	3 oz.	85	136	21.6	0.0	4.8
Trout (baked)	3 oz.	85	168	20.1	0.3	9.6
Tuna (cnd. in oil, drained)	3 oz.	85	170	24.0	0.0	7.0
Tuna (cnd. in water)	½ cup	100	127	28.0	0.0	0.8
Tuna salad	1 cup	205	350	30.0	7.0	22.0

FRUITS

Food	Amount	Weight (g)	Calories	Protein (g)	Carbohydrate (g)	Fat (g)
Apple, raw, with peel (2¾" diameter)	1 apple	138	80	0.0	20.0	1.0
Apple juice (bottled or cnd.)	1 cup	248	120	0.0	30.0	0.0
Applesauce, swt. (cnd.)	1 cup	255	230	1.0	61.0	0.0
Apricot nectar (cnd.)	1 cup	251	145	1.0	37.0	0.0
Apricots, dried (uncooked)	1 cup	130	340	7.0	86.0	1.0
Apricots, in heavy syrup (cnd.)	1 cup	258	220	2.0	57.0	0.0
Apricots, raw, without pits	3 apricots	107	55	1.0	14.0	0.0
Avocado, Florida	1 avocado	304	390	4.0	27.0	33.0
Banana	1 banana (medium)	119	100	1.0	26.0	0.0
Blackberries, fresh	1 cup	144	85	2.0	19.0	1.0
Blueberries, fresh	1 cup	145	90	1.0	22.0	1.0
Cantaloupe	½ melon	477	80	2.0	20.0	0.0
Cherries, fresh, sweet	10 cherries	68	45	1.0	12.0	0.0
Cranberry juice (bottled)	1 cup	253	165	0.0	42.0	0.0

FRUITS (Continued)

Food	Amount	Weight (g)	Calories	Protein (g)	Carbohydrate (g)	Fat (g)
Cranberry sauce, sweet (cnd.)	1 cup	277	405	0.0	104.0	1.0
Dates, whole, without pits	10 dates	80	220	2.0	58.0	0.0
Fruit cocktail (cnd.)	1 cup	255	195	1.0	50.0	0.0
Grape drink (cnd.)	1 cup	250	135	0.0	35.0	0.0
Grape juice (cnd. or bottled)	1 cup	253	165	1.0	42.0	0.0
Grapefruit, pink or red	½ grapefruit	241	50	1.0	13.0	0.0
Grapefruit, solids and liquid (cnd.)	1 cup	254	180	2.0	45.0	0.0
Grapefruit, white	½ grapefruit	241	45	1.0	12.0	0.0
Grapefruit juice, pink	1 cup	246	95	1.0	23.0	0.0
Grapefruit juice, unswt. (cnd.)	1 cup	247	100	1.0	24.0	0.0
Grapes, Thompson	10 grapes	50	35	0.0	9.0	0.0
Grapes, Tokay or Emperor	10 grapes	60	40	0.0	10.0	0.0
Guava	1 guava (medium)	100	62	0.8	15.0	0.6
Honeydew	⅒ melon	226	50	1.0	11.0	0.0
Lemon	1 lemon	74	20	1.0	6.0	0.0

FRUITS (Continued)

Food	Amount	Weight (g)	Calories	Protein (g)	Carbohydrate (g)	Fat (g)
Lemon juice	1 cup	244	60	1.0	20.0	0.0
Lemonade (from froz.)	1 cup	248	105	0.0	28.0	0.0
Lime juice	1 cup	246	65	1.0	22.0	0.0
Mango	½ mango (medium)	100	66	0.7	16.8	0.4
Orange, all varieties	1 orange	131	65	1.0	16.0	0.0
Orange juice	1 cup	248	110	2.0	26.0	0.0
Orange juice (from froz.)	1 cup	249	120	2.0	29.0	0.0
Orange juice, unswt. (cnd.)	1 cup	249	120	2.0	28.0	0.0
Orange/ grapefruit juice (from froz.)	1 cup	248	110	1.0	26.0	0.0
Papaya	1 cup	140	55	1.0	14.0	0.0
Peach, whole	1 peach	100	40	1.0	10.0	0.0
Peaches, dried, uncooked	1 cup	160	420	5.0	109.0	1.0
Peaches, heavy syrup (cnd.)	1 cup	256	200	1.0	51.0	0.0
Peaches, water pack	1 cup	244	75	1.0	20.0	0.0
Pear, Bartlett, with skin	1 pear	164	100	1.0	25.0	1.0
Pear, Bosco, with skin	1 pear	141	85	1.0	22.0	1.0
Pear, D'Anjou, with skin	1 pear	200	120	1.0	31.0	1.0

FRUITS (Continued)

Food	Amount	Weight (g)	Calories	Protein (g)	Carbohydrate (g)	Fat (g)
Pears, heavy syrup (cnd.)	1 cup	255	195	1.0	50.0	1.0
Persimmon, Japanese	1 medium persimmon	100	77	0.7	19.7	0.4
Persimmon, Japanese	1 medium persimmon	100	77	0.7	19.7	0.4
Pineapple, fresh, diced	1 cup	155	80	1.0	21.0	0.0
Pineapple, syrup bits (cnd.)	1 cup	255	190	1.0	20.0	0.0
Pineapple, syrup, large pieces (cnd.)	1 slice	105	80	0.0	20.0	0.0
Pineapple juice, unswt. (cnd.)	1 cup	250	140	1.0	34.0	0.0
Plum, fresh, Japanese or hybrid	1 plum	66	30	0.0	8.0	0.0
Plum, fresh, prune type	1 plum	28	20	0.0	6.0	0.0
Plums, heavy syrup (cnd.)	3 plums	140	110	1.0	29.0	0.0
Prune juice (cnd. or bottled)	1 cup	256	195	1.0	49.0	0.0
Raisins, seedless	1 cup	145	420	4.0	112.0	0.0
Raisins, seedless (packet)	½ oz.	14	40	0.0	1.0	0.0

FRUITS (Continued)

Food	Amount	Weight (g)	Calories	Protein (g)	Carbohydrate (g)	Fat (g)
Raspberries, red, fresh	1 cup	123	70	1.0	17.0	1.0
Raspberries, swt. (froz.)	10 oz.	284	280	2.0	70.0	1.0
Rhubarb (froz., swt.)	1 cup	270	385	1.0	98.0	1.0
Strawberries, fresh, whole	1 cup	149	55	1.0	13.0	1.0
Strawberries, sweet (froz.)	10 oz.	284	310	1.0	79.0	1.0
Strawberries, whole (froz.)	1¾ cup	454	415	2.0	107.0	1.0
Tangerine, no peel	1	86	40	1.0	10.0	0.0
Tangerine juice; sweet (cnd.)	1 cup	249	125	1.0	30.0	0.0
Watermelon	½ cup cubes	100	26	0.5	6.4	0.2
Watermelon, with rind	1 wedge	926	110	2.0	27.0	1.0

GRAINS

Food	Amount	Weight (g)	Calories	Protein (g)	Carbohydrate (g)	Fat (g)
Bagel, water	1 bagel	55	165	6.0	30.0	1.0
Barley, pearled, uncooked	1 cup	200	700	16.0	158.0	2.0

GRAINS (Continued)

Food	Amount	Weight (g)	Calories	Protein (g)	Carbohydrate (g)	Fat (g)
Biscuit (home recipe)	1 biscuit	28	105	2.0	13.0	5.0
Biscuit (mix)	1 biscuit	28	90	2.0	15.0	3.0
Bread, cracked wheat	1 slice	25	65	2.0	13.0	1.0
Bread, French, enr.	1 slice	35	100	3.0	19.0	1.0
Bread, Italian, enr.	1 slice	30	85	3.0	17.0	0.0
Bread, pumpernickel	1 slice	32	80	3.0	17.0	0.0
Bread, raisin, enr.	1 slice	25	65	200.0	13.0	1.0
Bread, rye, light	1 slice	25	60	2.0	13.0	0.0
Bread, wheat, firm	1 slice	25	60	3.0	12.0	1.0
Bread, white, soft	1 slice	25	70	2.0	13.0	1.0
Bread crumbs, dry, grated	1 cup	100	390	13.0	73.0	5.0
Bread crumbs, soft white	1 cup	45	120	4.0	23.0	1.0
Cake, angelfood	1/12 cake	53	135	3.0	32.0	0.0
Cake, Boston cream (home recipe)	1/12 cake	69	210	3.0	34.0	6.0
Cake, coffee (mix)	1/6 cake	72	230	5.0	38.0	7.0
Cake, cupcake, chocolate icing	1 cupcake	36	130	2.0	21.0	5.0

G R A I N S (Continued)

Food	Amount	Weight (g)	Calories	Protein (g)	Carbohydrate (g)	Fat (g)
Cake, cupcake, no icing	1 cupcake	25	90	1.0	14.0	3.0
Cake, cupcake, devil's food, icing	1 cupcake	35	120	2.0	20.0	4.0
Cake, devil's food, icing	1/16 cake	69	235	3.0	40.0	8.0
Cake, fruit, dark (home recipe)	1 loaf	454	1720	22.0	271.0	69.0
Cake, fruit, dark (home recipe)	1 slice = 1/11 of loaf	40	156	2.0	25.0	6.0
Cake, sponge (home recipe)	1/12 cake	66	195	5.0	36.0	4.0
Cereal, bran flakes 40% (generic)	3/4 cup	26	79	3.0	21.0	7.0
Cereal, bran with raisins	3/4 cup	38	109	3.0	30.0	1.0
Cereal, Cheerios, (General Mills)	3/4 cup	19	73	3.0	13.0	1.0
Cereal, corn flakes	3/4 cup	19	71	2.0	16.0	0.0
Cereal, corn flakes with sugar	3/4 cup	30	116	2.0	28.0	0.0
Cereal, corn grits, unenr.	3/4 cup	184	94	2.0	20.0	0.0

GRAINS (Continued)

Food	Amount	Weight (g)	Calories	Protein (g)	Carbohydrate (g)	Fat (g)
Cereal, corn Total, (General Mills)	¾ cup	21	82	1.5	17.8	0.0
Cereal, Farina, unenr.	¾ cup	184	79	2.0	16.0	0.0
Cereal, granola, Pillsbury	¾ cup	84	360	9.0	57.0	12.0
Cereal, oatmeal	¾ cup	180	98	4.0	17.0	2.0
Cereal, puffed corn	1 cup	20	80	2.0	16.0	1.0
Cereal, puffed oats	1 cup	25	100	3.0	19.0	1.0
Cereal, puffed rice	1 cup	15	60	1.0	13.0	0.0
Cereal, puffed wheat	1 cup	15	55	2.0	12.0	0.0
Cereal, shredded wheat	¾ cup	19	68	2.0	15.0	1.0
Cereal, wheat flakes	¾ cup	22	79	2.0	18.0	0.0
Cereal, wheat germ	1 tbs.	6	25	2.0	3.0	1.0
Cereal, wheat (rolled)	¾ cup	180	135	4.0	31.0	1.0
Cookie, brownies (mix)	1 brownie	20	85	1.0	13.0	4.0
Cookie, chocolate chip (mix)	4 cookies	42	200	2.0	29.0	9.0

GRAINS *(Continued)*

Food	Amount	Weight (g)	Calories	Protein (g)	Carbohydrate (g)	Fat (g)
Cookie, fig bars	4 cookies	56	200	2.0	42.0	3.0
Cookie, ginger snaps	4 cookies	28	90	2.0	22.0	2.0
Cookie, macaroons	2 cookies	38	180	2.0	25.0	9.0
Cookie, oatmeal with raisins	4 cookies	52	235	3.0	38.0	8.0
Crackers, graham, plain	2 crackers	14	55	1.0	10.0	1.0
Crackers, rye wafers	2 wafers	13	45	2.0	10.0	0.0
Crackers, Saltines	4 crackers	11	50	1.0	8.0	1.0
Crackers, sesame	4 crackers	12	60	7.3	1.2	2.9
Danish pastry, plain	1 ring	340	1435	25.0	155.0	80.0
Danish pastry, plain	1 pastry	65	275	5.0	30.0	15.0
Doughnut, cake, plain	1 doughnut	25	100	1.0	13.0	5.0
Doughnut, yeast, glazed	1 doughnut	50	205	3.0	22.0	11.0
Flour (wheat), cake, sifted	1 cup	96	350	7.0	76.0	1.0
Flour (wheat), enr., sifted	1 cup	115	420	12.0	88.0	1.0
Flour (wheat), enr., unsifted	1 cup	125	455	13.0	95.0	1.0
Flour (wheat), self-rising	1 cup	125	440	12.0	93.0	1.0

GRAINS (Continued)

Food	Amount	Weight (g)	Calories	Protein (g)	Carbohydrate (g)	Fat (g)
Flour (wheat), whole, hard	1 cup	120	400	16.0	85.0	2.0
Macaroni (cooked, firm)	1 cup	130	190	7.0	39.0	1.0
Macaroni and cheese (cnd.)	1 cup	240	230	9.0	26.0	10.0
Macaroni and cheese (home recipe)	1 cup	200	430	17.0	40.0	22.0
Muffin, blueberry (home recipe)	1 small muffin	40	110	3.0	17.0	4.0
Muffin, bran (home recipe)	1 small muffin	40	105	3.0	17.0	4.0
Muffin, corn (home recipe)	1 small muffin	40	125	3.0	19.0	4.0
Muffin, corn (mix, egg and milk)	1 small muffin	40	130	3.0	20.0	4.0
Muffin, plain (home recipe)	1 small muffin	40	120	3.0	17.0	4.0
Noodles, chow mein (cnd.)	1 cup	45	220	6.0	26.0	11.0
Noodles, egg, enr. (cooked)	1 cup	160	200	7.0	37.0	2.0
Pancake, buckwheat (mix)	1 cake	27	55	2.0	6.0	2.0
Pancake, plain (home recipe)	1 cake	27	60	2.0	9.0	2.0
Pancake, plain (mix)	1 cake	27	60	2.0	9.0	2.0

G R A I N S (Continued)

Food	Amount	Weight (g)	Calories	Protein (g)	Carbohydrate (g)	Fat (g)
Pie, apple	1 average slice	135	345	3.0	51.0	15.0
Pie, banana cream	1 average slice	130	285	6.0	40.0	12.0
Pie, blueberry	1 average slice	135	325	3.0	47.0	15.0
Pie, cherry	1 average slice	135	350	4.0	52.0	15.0
Pie, custard	1 average slice	130	285	8.0	30.0	14.0
Pie, lemon meringue	1 average slice	120	305	4.0	45.0	12.0
Pie, mince	1 average slice	135	365	3.0	56.0	16.0
Pie, peach	1 average slice	135	345	3.0	52.0	14.0
Pie, pecan	1 average slice	118	495	6.0	61.0	27.0
Pie, pumpkin	1 average slice	130	275	5.0	32.0	15.0
Pie crust, baked (mix)	2 shells	320	1485	20.0	141.0	93.0
Pizza, cheese (baked)	1 average slice	100	225	11	25	9
Popcorn, plain (popped)	1 cup	6	25	1.0	5.0	0.0
Popcorn, with oil and salt	1 cup	9	40	1.0	5.0	2.0
Pretzels, stick	10 pretzels	3	10	0.0	2.0	0.0
Pretzels, twisted	10 pretzels	60	235	6.0	46.0	3.0
Rice, brown	1 cup	150	178	4.0	38.0	1.0
Rice, white, instant, (cooked)	1 cup	165	180	4.0	40.0	0.0
Rice, white, long-grain (cooked)	1 cup	205	225	4.0	50.0	0.0
Roll, brown and serve, enr.	1 roll	26	85	2.0	14.0	2.0

GRAINS (Continued)

Food	Amount	Weight (g)	Calories	Protein (g)	Carbohydrate (g)	Fat (g)
Roll, frankfurter or hamburger	1 roll	40	120	3.0	21.0	2.0
Roll, hard, enr.	1 roll	50	155	5.0	30.0	2.0
Roll, hoagie or submarine, enr.	1 roll	135	390	12.0	75.0	4.0
Spaghetti (cooked, firm)	1 cup	130	190	7.0	39.0	1.0
Spaghetti (cooked, tender)	1 cup	140	155	5.0	32.0	1.0
Spaghetti, tomato and cheese (cnd.)	1 cup	250	190	6.0	39.0	2.0
Spaghetti, tomato and meat (cnd.)	1 cup	250	260	12.0	29.0	10.0
Waffle, enr. (home recipe)	1 waffle	75	210	7.0	28.0	7.0
Waffle, enr. (mix, egg and milk)	1 waffle	75	205	7.0	27.0	8.0

MEAT AND POULTRY

Food	Amount	Weight (g)	Calories	Protein (g)	Carbohydrate (g)	Fat (g)
Bacon (broiled or fried, crisp)	2 slices	15	85	4.0	0.0	8.0
Beef, ground, choice grade (30% fat)	3 oz.	86	213	25.0	0.0	12.0
Beef, roast, rib, L & F (broiled)	3 oz.	85	375	17.0	0.0	33.0
Beef, round, heel, L & F (roasted)	3 oz.	85	190	27.0	0.0	8.0
Beef, L & F (simmered or roasted)	3 oz.	85	245	23.0	0.0	16.0
Beef, sirloin steak, L & F (broiled)	3 oz.	85	330	20.0	0.0	27.0
Beef and vegetable stew	1 cup	245	220	16.0	15.0	11.0
Beef pot pie (home recipe)	⅓ pie	210	515	21.0	39.0	30.0
Bologna	1 slice	28	85	3.0	0.0	8.0
Chicken (broiled)	6.2 oz.	176	240	42.0	0.0	7.0
Chicken, boneless (canned)	3 oz.	85	170	18.0	0.0	10.0
Chicken, light meat, no skin (roasted)	3½ oz.	100	166	31.6	0.0	3.4
Chicken breast (broiled)	3½ oz.	100	136	23.8	0.0	3.8
Chicken breast (fried)	½ breast	79	160	26.0	1.0	5.0
Chicken drumstick (fried)	1.3 oz.	38	90	12.0	0	4.0
Chili con carne (canned)	1 cup	255	340	19.0	31	16.0
Duck, domestic, no skin (roasted)	3½ oz.	100	310	22.8	0.0	23.6
Frankfurter (cooked)	1 frank	56	170	7.0	1.0	15.0

MEAT AND POULTRY (Continued)

Food	Amount	Weight (g)	Calories	Protein (g)	Carbohydrate (g)	Fat (g)
Frog legs (raw)	3½ oz.	100	73	16.4	0.0	0.2
Frog legs (fried)	3½ oz.	100	290	17.9	8.5	19.8
Ham, boiled, luncheon	1 slice	28	65	5.0	0.0	5.0
Ham, L & F (roasted)	3 oz.	85	245	18.0	0.0	19.0
Lamb chop, rib, L & F (broiled)	3.1 oz.	89	360	18.0	0.0	32.0
Lamb, leg, L & F (roasted)	3 oz.	85	235	22.0	0.0	16.0
Lamb, shoulder, L & F (roasted)	3 oz.	85	285	18.0	0.0	23.0
Liver, beef (fried)	3 oz.	85	195	22.0	5.0	9.0
Pork chop, loin, L & F (broiled)	2.7 oz.	78	305	19.0	0.0	25.0
Pork roast, L & F (oven cooked)	3 oz.	85	310	21.0	0.0	24.0
Pork shoulder, L & F (roasted)	3 oz.	85	320	20.0	0.0	26.0
Pork shoulder, lean (roasted)	2.2 oz.	63	135	18.0	0.0	6.0
Salami, cooked type	1 oz.	28	90	5.0	0.0	7.0
Salami, dry type	⅓ oz.	10	45	2.0	0.0	4.0
Sausage, pork link	1 link	13	60	2.0	0.0	6.0
Turkey, dark meat, no skin	4 pieces	85	175	26.0	0.0	7.0
Turkey, light meat, no skin	2 pieces	85	150	28.0	0.0	3.0
Veal cutlet, L & F (cooked)	3 oz.	85	216	26.0	0.0	12.0
Veal, ribs, no bone (roasted)	3 oz.	85	230	23.0	0.0	14.0
Venison (raw)	3½ oz.	100	124	21.4	0.0	3.6

NUTS, SEEDS, AND LEGUMES

Food	Amount	Weight (g)	Calories	Protein (g)	Carbohydrate (g)	Fat (g)
Almonds, shelled, chopped	1 cup	130	775	24.0	25.0	70.0
Almonds, shelled, slivered	1 cup	115	690	21.0	22.0	62.0
Beans, Great North, dry (cooked)	1 cup	180	210	14.0	38.0	1.0
Beans, Navy Pea, dry (cooked)	1 cup	190	225	15.0	40.0	1.0
Brazil nuts, shelled	1 oz.	28	185	4.0	3.0	19.0
Cashew nuts (roasted in oil)	1 cup	140	785	24.0	41.0	64.0
Coconut meat, fresh	1 piece	45	155	2.0	4.0	16.0
Coconut meat, fresh, shredded	1 cup	80	275	3.0	8.0	28.0
Filberts, chopped	1 cup	115	730	14.0	19.0	72.0
Lentils, whole (cooked)	1 cup	200	210	16.0	39.0	0.0
Peanut butter	1 tbs.	16	95	4.0	3.0	8.0
Peanuts (roasted with oil and salt)	1 cup	144	840	37.0	27.0	72.0
Peas, split, dry (cooked)	1 cup	200	230	16.0	42.0	1.0
Pecans, chopped or pieces	1 cup	118	810	11.0	17.0	84.0
Pumpkin / squash seeds, dry	1 cup	140	775	41.0	21.0	65.0
Sunflower seeds, dry	1 cup	145	810	35.0	29.0	69.0

NUTS, SEEDS, AND LEGUMES (Continued)

Food	Amount	Weight (g)	Calories	Protein (g)	Carbohydrate (g)	Fat (g)
Walnuts, black, chopped	1 cup	125	785	26.0	19.0	74.0
Walnuts, black, fine ground	1 cup	80	500	16.0	12.0	47.0
Walnuts, black, whole	4–5 (whole)	15	94	3.0	3.0	9.0

SWEETS

Food	Amount	Weight (g)	Calories	Protein (g)	Carbohydrate (g)	Fat (g)
Candy, caramels, plain or chocolate	1 oz. (3 pieces)	28	115	1.0	22.0	3.0
Candy, milk chocolate	1 oz.	28	145	2.0	16.0	9.0
Candy, chocolate coated peanuts	1 oz.	28	160	5.0	11.0	12.0
Candy, fudge chocolate	1 oz.	28	115	1.0	21.0	3.0
Candy, Hershey Kit Kat bar	1 bar	35	180	2.5	21.5	9.3
Candy, marsh-mallows	1 oz.	28	90	1.0	23.0	0.0
Chocolate chips, Nestle, semi-sweet	1 oz.	28	148	1.0	17.8	7.9
Honey	1 tbs.	21	65	0.0	17.0	0.0
Jams (all varieties)	1 tbs.	20	55	0.0	14.0	0.0

VEGETABLES

Food	Amount	Weight (g)	Calories	Protein (g)	Carbohydrate (g)	Fat (g)
Asparagus spears (cnd.)	4 spears	80	15	2.0	3.0	0.0
Asparagus spears	4 spears	60	10	1.0	2.0	0.0
Asparagus tips	1 cup	145	30	3.0	5.0	0.0
Bean sprouts, Mung, fresh	1 cup	105	35	4.0	7.0	0.0
Bean sprouts, Mung (cooked)	1 cup	125	35	4.0	7.0	0.0
Beans, lima, thick (cooked from froz.)	1 cup	170	170	10.0	32.0	0.0
Beans, lima, thin (cooked from froz.)	1 cup	180	210	13.0	40.0	0.0
Beans, snap, green	1 cup	130	30	2.0	7.0	0.0
Beans, snap, wax (cooked or raw)	1 cup	125	30	2.0	6.0	0.0
Beans, snap, yellow or wax (froz. or cnd.)	1 cup	135	35	2.0	8.0	0.0
Beet greens (cooked, drained)	1 cup	145	25	2.0	5.0	0.0
Beets, peeled, sliced (cooked)	1 cup	170	55	2.0	12.0	0.0
Beets, peeled, whole (cooked)	2 beets	100	30	1.0	7.0	0.0
Beets, sliced (cnd., drained)	1 cup	170	65	2.0	15.0	0.0
Beets, whole (cnd., drained)	1 cup	160	60	2.0	14.0	0.0
Broccoli (cooked or raw)	1 stalk	180	45	6.0	8.0	1.0

VEGETABLES (Continued)

Food	Amount	Weight (g)	Calories	Protein (g)	Carbohydrate (g)	Fat (g)
Broccoli (cooked or raw)	1 cup	155	40	5.0	7.0	0.0
Broccoli (cooked from froz.)	1 stalk	30	10	1.0	1.0	0.0
Broccoli (cooked from froz.)	1 cup	185	50	5.0	9.0	1.0
Brussels sprouts (cooked or raw)	1 cup	155	55	7.0	10.0	1.0
Brussels sprouts (cooked from froz.)	1 cup	155	50	5.0	10.0	0.0
Cabbage, common, raw, shredded	1 cup	90	20	1.0	5.0	0.0
Cabbage, common, raw, sliced	1 cup	70	15	1.0	4.0	0.0
Cabbage, red, sliced	1 cup	140	30	3.0	6.0	0.0
Carrot, raw, grated	1 cup	110	45	1.0	11.0	0.0
Carrot, raw, scraped	1 carrot	72	30	1.0	7.0	0.0
Carrot, sliced (cnd., drained)	1 cup	155	45	1.0	10.0	0.0
Cauliflower	1 cup	140	30	3.0	6.0	0.0
Celery, Pascal type, raw	1 stalk	40	5	0.0	2.0	0.0
Collards (cooked or raw, drained)	1 cup	190	65	7.0	10.0	1.0
Collards (cooked from froz., drained)	1 cup	170	50	5.0	10.0	1.0
Corn, sweet (cooked or raw, drained)	1 ear	140	70	2.0	16.0	1.0

VEGETABLES (Continued)

Food	Amount	Weight (g)	Calories	Protein (g)	Carbohydrate (g)	Fat (g)
Corn, sweet (cooked from froz., drained)	1 ear	229	120	4.0	27.0	1.0
Corn, sweet (cooked from froz., drained)	1 cup	165	130	5.0	31.0	1.0
Corn, sweet, cream style (cnd.)	1 cup	256	210	5.0	51.0	2.0
Corn, sweet, vacuum pack (cnd.)	1 cup	210	175	5.0	43.0	1.0
Corn, sweet, wet pack (cnd.)	1 cup	165	140	4.0	33.0	1.0
Cucumber, with peel	6–8 slices	28	5	0.0	1.0	0.0
Endive, curly (escarole)	1 cup	50	10	1.0	2.0	0.0
Kale (cooked or raw, drained)	1 cup	110	45	5.0	7.0	1.0
Kale (cooked from froz., drained)	1 cup	130	40	4.0	7.0	1.0
Lettuce, butterhead (raw)	1 head	220	25	2.0	4.0	0.0
Lettuce, butterhead (raw)	2 leaves	15	0	0.0	0.0	0.0
Lettuce, iceberg (raw)	1 head	567	70	5.0	16.0	0.0
Lettuce, iceberg (raw)	¼ head	135	20	1.0	4.0	0.0
Lettuce, looseleaf (raw)	1 cup	55	10	1.0	2.0	0.0
Mushrooms, chopped (raw)	1 cup	70	20	2.0	3.0	0.0
Okra pods (cooked)	10 pods	106	30	2.0	6.0	0.0

VEGETABLES (Continued)

Food	Amount	Weight (g)	Calories	Protein (g)	Carbohydrate (g)	Fat (g)
Onions, mature, chopped (raw)	1 cup	170	65	3.0	15.0	0.0
Onions, mature, sliced (raw)	1 cup	115	45	2.0	10.0	0.0
Onions, mature (cooked, drained)	1 cup	210	60	3.0	14.0	0.0
Onions, young green	6 onions	30	15	0.0	3.0	0.0
Parsley, chopped (raw)	1 tbs.	4	0	0.0	0.0	0.0
Parsnips (cooked)	1 cup	155	100	2.0	23.0	1.0
Peas, green (cooked from froz., drained)	1 cup	160	110	8.0	19.0	0.0
Peas, green, whole (cnd.)	1 cup	170	150	8.0	29.0	1.0
Peppers, sweet (raw)	1 pod	74	15	1.0	4.0	0.0
Peppers, sweet (boiled)	1 pod	73	15	1.0	3.0	0.0
Potato (baked, peeled after)	1 potato	135	100	4.0	33.0	0.0
Potato (boiled, peeled after)	1 potato	137	105	3.0	23.0	0.0
Potato (boiled, peeled before)	1 potato	135	90	3.0	20.0	0.0
Potato, hash brown (cooked from froz.)	1 cup	155	345	3.0	45.0	18.0
Potato, mashed (milk)	1 cup	210	135	4.0	27.0	2.0
Potato, mashed (milk and butter)	1 cup	210	195	4.0	26.0	9.0
Potato chips	10 chips	20	115	1.0	10.0	8.0
Potato salad	1 cup	250	250	7.0	41.0	7.0

VEGETABLES (Continued)

Food	Amount	Weight (g)	Calories	Protein (g)	Carbohydrate (g)	Fat (g)
Pumpkin (cnd.)	1 cup	245	80	2.0	19.0	1.0
Radishes (raw)	4 radishes	18	5	0.0	1.0	0.0
Sauerkraut (cnd.)	1 cup	235	40	2.0	9.0	0.0
Spinach, chopped (raw)	1 cup	55	15	2.0	2.0	0.0
Spinach (cooked, drained)	1 cup	180	40	5.0	6.0	1.0
Squash, summer (cooked, diced)	1 cup	210	30	2.0	7.0	0.0
Squash, winter (baked, mashed)	1 cup	205	130	4.0	32.0	1.0
Sweet potato (baked, peeled)	1 potato	114	160	2.0	37.0	1.0
Sweet potato (boiled, peeled)	1 potato	151	170	3.0	40.0	1.0
Tofu	3½ oz.	100	72	7.8	2.4	4.2
Tomato (raw)	1 tomato	135	25	1.0	6.0	0.0
Tomato (cnd., solids and liquid)	1 cup	241	50	2.0	10.0	0.0
Tomato catsup	1 cup	273	290	5.0	69.0	1.0
Tomato catsup	1 tbs.	15	15	0.0	4.0	0.0
Tomato juice (cnd.)	1 cup	243	45	2.0	10.0	0.0
Turnip greens, whole (cooked from fresh)	1 cup	145	30	3.0	5.0	0.0
Turnip greens, chopped (cooked from froz.)	1 cup	165	40	4.0	6.0	0.0
Turnips (cooked, diced)	1 cup	155	35	1.0	8.0	0.0
Vegetables, mixed (cooked from froz.)	1 cup	182	115	6.0	24.0	1.0

MISCELLANEOUS

Food	Amount	Weight (g)	Calories	Protein (g)	Carbohydrate (g)	Fat (g)
Beef pot pie, commercial froz.	1 pie	227	443	16.6	37.0	25.4
Beef stew, Sara Lee froz.	1 portion	200	304	45.0	8.0	8.6
Chicken à la King, Weight Watchers	1 serving	256	230	26.0	15.0	7.0
Egg roll, chicken, La Choy froz.	1 egg roll	100	242	8.1	29.4	10.2
Ham dinner, Morton froz.	1 dinner	283	429	18.5	49.1	18.1
Mustard, brown	1 tsp.	5	4	0.3	0.3	0.4
Pizza, cheese, homemade	1 slice (5⅓" arch)	65	145	2.7	23.7	4.4
Taco with beef and cheese	1 average taco	75	162	11.8	8.9	8.6
White sauce, medium	¼ cup	66	107	2.6	6.1	8.1

Index

214 • Index

CHECK
W/ HOSPITAL
CHECK ARSON
M—

ALSO CHECK
MY UNDERARM
O WRIST

RIVVER

HUDSON
PHILIP ARMY

HELD IN
IN HELD
MARK

HERE'S HOW...

HOW TO BUY A CAR by James R. Ross
The essential guide that gives you the edge in buying a new or used car.
_____ 90198-4 $3.95 U.S.   _____ 90199-2 $4.95 Can.

THE WHOLESALE-BY-MAIL CATALOG—UPDATE 1986 by The Print Project
Everything you need at 30% to 90% off retail prices—by mail or phone!
_____ 90379-0 $3.95 U.S.   _____ 90380-4 $4.95 Can.

TAKING CARE OF CLOTHES: An Owner's Manual for Care, Repair and Spot Removal by Mablen Jones
The most comprehensive handbook of its kind...save money—and save your wardrobe!
_____ 90355-0 $4.95 U.S.   _____ 90356-1 $6.25 Can.

AND THE LUCKY WINNER IS...The Complete Guide to Winning Sweepstakes & Contests
by Carolyn and Roger Tyndall with Tad Tuleja
Increase the odds in your favor—all you need to know.
_____ 90025-2 $3.95 U.S.   _____ 90026-0 $4.95 Can.

THE OFFICIAL HARVARD STUDENT AGENCIES BARTENDING COURSE
The new complete guide to drinkmaking—the $40 course now a paperback book!
_____ 90427-4 $3.95 U.S.   _____ 90430-4 $4.95 Can.